You don't need perfection to make progress
— only the courage to begin. So let's begin.

Table of Contents

The Freitas Weight Loss Method

Part One

1. Presentation of the Concept – The Freitas Method

Weight loss is a deeply personal journey. For many, it's a cycle of short-term success followed by frustration and relapse. Diets come and go, but lasting change only happens when we shift our daily behaviors and mindset. That's where the Freitas Method comes in. The Freitas Method is not a diet. It doesn't tell you what to eat or forbid certain foods. Instead, it introduces a structured scoring system that helps you build awareness, create daily discipline, and reinforce positive habits — regardless of which eating style or weight loss approach you follow.

This method was born from a simple observation: we often know what we should do to lose weight, but we lack the tools to consistently apply that knowledge in real life. By translating your daily actions — what you eat, how you move, how much water you drink — into a daily score, the Freitas Method gives you immediate feedback, direction, and motivation.

Just like athletes use stats to improve their performance, you'll use your score to track your own progress — not just in weight, but in behavior. The Freitas Method encourages gradual, sustainable change. It transforms the abstract goal of "losing weight" into tangible, achievable actions you can repeat every day.

This book is divided into three parts. The first part explains the Freitas Method in depth, along with the psychological and behavioral principles behind it, as well as essential concepts of nutrition, diet types, and the science of weight loss. Reading this section is important to give you a solid foundation and ensure you apply the method in the second part with clarity and confidence.

The second part of the book presents the scoring criteria and guidelines — explaining how each habit is evaluated.

The third part is the practical section, where you'll apply this system through daily logs and weekly tracking, turning knowledge into consistent action.

This book will show you how to apply the method, understand your results, and use the system to stay engaged and on track — for the long term.

2. The Freitas Method is Not a Diet

In a world overflowing with diet trends, meal plans, and food rules, it's easy to get overwhelmed. Many people jump from one diet to another, searching for the "perfect" one — only to feel discouraged when results don't last. The truth is: there is no universal diet that works for everyone.

That's why the Freitas Method takes a different path. It's not a diet — it's a system. It doesn't prescribe a specific way of eating. Instead, it enhances whatever diet you choose to follow by introducing a daily scoring system that promotes self-awareness, consistency, and accountability.

Whether you're on a ketogenic diet, intermittent fasting, plant-based eating, or simply aiming for balanced nutrition, the Freitas Method fits right in. It doesn't compete with your diet — it supports it.

This flexibility is one of the method's greatest strengths. Instead of locking you into rigid rules, it gives you a tool to evaluate and improve your daily decisions, no matter the dietary approach. That way, the focus shifts from perfection to progress. You stop asking "Did I break the rules today?" and start asking "How well did I support my goals today?"

The Freitas Method respects your autonomy. It empowers you to make adjustments that fit your lifestyle, preferences, and challenges — while still holding you accountable in a positive, structured way.

Ultimately, it's not about following a diet perfectly. It's about creating a lifestyle that helps you succeed sustainably.

It also reduces the emotional pressure often associated with dieting, replacing guilt with curiosity and reflection. Instead of labeling foods as "good" or "bad," you begin to see patterns, choices, and areas for improvement. Over time, this builds confidence and trust in your own decision-making. The method is designed to support long-term behavioral change, not quick fixes. In that sense, it acts as a bridge between nutritional knowledge and daily execution — the part where most diets fail.

3. Applicable to Any Type of Diet

One of the core strengths of the Freitas Method is its adaptability. This system is not bound to a specific nutritional philosophy. Instead, it can be layered over any diet you choose to follow, acting as a powerful reinforcement tool — not a replacement.

Whether you're trying: Ketogenic – Low carb, high fat; Low-Carb – Moderate reduction in carbohydrates; Mediterranean – Whole foods, healthy fats, and lean proteins; Paleolithic (Paleo) – Focus on ancestral, unprocessed foods; Plant-Based or Vegan – Emphasis on plant sources and exclusion of animal products; Intermittent Fasting – Structured eating windows; DASH Diet – Designed for heart health and blood pressure control; Flexible or Calorie Counting – Macro-based or portion-focused eating ...the Freitas Method can support your goals.

It does this by focusing not on what you eat, but on how consistently you follow your chosen path. The daily scoring structure is centered on behaviors — such as the quality of your meals, hydration, and physical activity — rather than prescribing menus or calorie limits.

This means the method works equally well whether you're working with a nutritionist, following an app, or self-managing your plan. It respects your dietary choices while providing a feedback loop that helps keep you on track.

By removing the pressure to follow a "one-size-fits-all" plan, the Freitas Method creates space for flexibility, personalization, and long-term success — the things most traditional diets fail to deliver.

It also allows for a smoother transition when changing dietary strategies. If you decide to shift from one approach to another — for example, moving from calorie counting to a Mediterranean plan, or trying intermittent fasting — the Freitas Method stays with you. Your scoring habits remain stable, offering continuity, structure, and motivation during times of adjustment. This helps prevent the common loss of momentum that occurs when switching diets.

Another advantage is its ability to highlight what's working and what isn't within your current plan. Over time, your score trends can reveal patterns: perhaps your nutrition is solid but your activity level is inconsistent, or maybe hydration is where you're losing points. This data-driven awareness makes it easier to make targeted improvements without needing to overhaul your entire approach.

Lastly, by being diet-agnostic, the Freitas Method can serve as a common tracking tool for people with different eating styles. Whether in a family or support group, it creates a shared system for monitoring progress — without requiring everyone to follow the same diet.

4. Differences and Similarities Between Diets

There are countless diet plans available, each claiming to be the best approach for weight loss. While there are numerous differences between them, they share key similarities — particularly when it comes to the fundamental principles of weight loss. The Freitas Method is not a diet itself, but rather a framework that can be applied to any diet, promoting consistency and helping individuals track their behaviors to achieve lasting weight loss.

Common Principles Across Diets

While the specifics may vary from one diet to another, all weight loss diets rely on a few core principles that are universally recognized in the science of nutrition:

Caloric Deficit: Regardless of the type of diet, all successful weight loss plans require creating a caloric deficit — burning more calories than you consume. Whether through portion control, food choices, or exercise, a calorie deficit is essential for fat loss.

Nutrient Quality: Many diets emphasize the importance of nutrient-dense foods, focusing on whole, minimally processed foods. These foods provide essential vitamins, minerals, and other nutrients while keeping calorie intake in check.

Macronutrient Balance: Most diets include guidelines for balancing macronutrients (carbohydrates, proteins, and fats) to support overall health, muscle maintenance, and fat loss. The exact proportions of these macronutrients will vary by diet, but each aims to optimize energy use and prevent nutrient deficiencies.

Sustainability: The most effective diets are those that promote long-term lifestyle changes, not quick fixes. Restrictive diets may show fast results but are often difficult to maintain over time, leading to weight regain. The Freitas Method, with its scoring system, supports this by encouraging gradual, sustainable changes rather than dramatic restrictions.

Examples of Popular Diets

To better understand how the Freitas Method can be applied to different approaches, let's look at some of the most common diets and how they align with these principles:

Low-Carb Diets (e.g., Keto, Atkins)
Main Principle: Low-carb diets focus on significantly reducing carbohydrate intake to shift the body into a state of ketosis (for Keto) or simply restrict carbs for fat loss.

Plant-Based Diets (e.g., Vegan, Vegetarian)
Main Principle: These diets emphasize plant-based foods and eliminate animal products, focusing on vegetables, fruits, legumes, and whole grains.

Intermittent Fasting (IF)
Main Principle: Intermittent fasting focuses on the timing of food intake rather than food types, typically alternating between periods of eating and fasting.

Mediterranean Diet
Main Principle: This diet emphasizes healthy fats (particularly from olive oil), lean proteins, whole grains, and a variety of fruits and vegetables. It has a focus on heart health and overall longevity.

Paleo Diet
Main Principle: The Paleo diet promotes eating foods that would have been available to our pre-agricultural ancestors, focusing on meat, fish, fruits, vegetables, nuts, and seeds. Processed foods, grains, and legumes are avoided

DASH Diet (Dietary Approaches to Stop Hypertension)
Main Principle: Originally designed to help lower blood pressure, the DASH diet emphasizes nutrient-dense foods such as fruits, vegetables, lean proteins, and low-fat dairy, while reducing sodium and processed foods. It's widely recommended for cardiovascular health.

Flexible Dieting / IIFYM (If It Fits Your Macros)
Main Principle: This approach allows for greater food freedom by focusing on meeting daily targets for macronutrients (proteins, carbs, fats), regardless of food source. It encourages balance and moderation rather than food restriction.

The Unifying Concept: Healthy Choices and Consistency

While each diet plan has its specific set of rules, the Freitas Method emphasizes a unifying principle: healthy choices and consistency lead to sustainable results. Regardless of the diet you choose to follow — whether it's low-carb, plant-based, intermittent fasting, or Mediterranean — the core concept remains the same. By tracking and scoring your daily actions, you can make informed decisions and adjust your behaviors to align with your goals.

While some flexible dieting approaches may allow for occasional indulgence, no serious or evidence-based diet promotes ice cream, soft drinks, cakes, or French fries as healthy choices. For this reason, the Freitas Method penalizes the consumption of such foods by reducing the points awarded, as they do not contribute to nutritional quality or long-term health goals.

The method isn't a "one-size-fits-all" approach; rather, it provides a flexible structure that supports any dietary plan. It helps individuals stay on track with their personal goals by focusing on the three pillars of weight loss: nutrition, hydration, and physical activity. It doesn't compete with other diets; it complements them. By integrating daily self-monitoring, it empowers individuals to create lasting habits that align with any dietary choice. Consistency and sustainable habits are the true keys to success in any weight loss journey.

The Freitas Method also emphasizes that consistency doesn't mean perfection. It's about making progress over time. You don't need to follow every rule to the letter every single day. Instead, it's about making informed, healthier choices more often than not. By using the scoring system, you can gradually build habits that support long-term success, allowing you to move past occasional setbacks and stay focused on your bigger goals.

Ultimately, the method encourages self-awareness and self-discipline, two crucial components for any sustainable weight loss or health journey. Whether you're managing your weight, improving fitness, or simply aiming for healthier living, the Freitas Method keeps you accountable without overwhelming you with rigid rules. It creates a balanced approach where health and enjoyment coexist, enabling you to stay committed to your diet and your overall well-being.

5. Psychological and Behavioral Foundations

Sustainable weight loss is not just about nutrition — it's about behavior. Many people know what to do, but they struggle with the how and the why. The Freitas Method is designed with this in mind. It incorporates basic principles from psychology and habit formation to help turn healthy intentions into consistent actions.

At the core of the method is the idea of self-monitoring. Studies show that simply tracking behavior increases awareness and leads to better outcomes. By scoring your daily habits, the Freitas Method creates a feedback loop that reinforces the behaviors you want to strengthen — whether it's eating better, moving more, or staying hydrated.

This scoring system taps into a natural human drive: the desire for progress. When you see your daily score, you're not just evaluating your diet — you're seeing a reflection of your effort and discipline. Over time, this builds motivation, self-efficacy, and consistency — all essential for lasting change.

The method also supports habit building. By encouraging daily repetition of small, healthy choices, it turns intentional behavior into automatic behavior. These micro-decisions, tracked and acknowledged, are the building blocks of transformation.

Importantly, the Freitas Method promotes self-compassion over self-judgment. A low score is not failure — it's feedback. It allows you to identify patterns, make adjustments, and keep moving forward without shame or guilt. In short, this method is as much about changing your mindset as it is about changing your meals.

In addition to self-monitoring, it encourages the development of intrinsic motivation — the desire to make healthy choices for the sake of personal well-being rather than external pressures. It shifts the focus away from quick fixes and temporary solutions and instead fosters a deeper connection to your goals. By gradually improving your score each day, you create a sense of accomplishment that builds a positive feedback loop, strengthening your commitment to healthy habits.

Moreover, the method understands that change is not linear. There will be days where you fall short of your goals, and that's okay. The Freitas Method helps you embrace setbacks as opportunities to learn and grow, rather than seeing them as failures. With the right mindset, even difficult days can propel you forward, as they offer insights into what adjustments are needed to continue progressing toward your goals. This approach ensures that your journey is sustainable, adaptable, and ultimately successful.

6. Theoretical Foundations of Weight Loss

Understanding the science behind weight loss is key to making informed decisions and setting realistic expectations. The Freitas Method is grounded in well-established principles of metabolism, energy balance, and nutrition. Here, we'll explore the core concepts that drive the method and explain why these concepts are crucial for sustainable weight loss.

Caloric Deficit: The Core Principle

At the heart of any weight loss strategy is the concept of the caloric deficit. This simply means that, to lose weight, you need to burn more calories than you consume. This energy imbalance forces the body to tap into its fat stores for fuel, leading to weight loss over time.
- *Calories In*: The energy you consume from food and drink.
- *Calories Out*: The energy you expend through physical activity, metabolism, and bodily functions.

The Freitas Method encourages the creation of a sustainable caloric deficit. Unlike extreme diets that drastically cut calories, this method promotes gradual changes that support consistent weight loss without sacrificing essential nutrients or energy.

Empty Calories vs. Nutrient-Dense Calories

Not all calories are created equal. While it's important to maintain a caloric deficit, it's equally important to consider the quality of those calories.

Empty calories come from foods that provide little to no nutritional value. These are typically processed foods, sugary drinks, and refined snacks that are high in calories but lack vitamins, minerals, and fiber.

Nutrient-dense calories, on the other hand, come from whole foods that are rich in essential nutrients. These foods provide your body with the vitamins, minerals, protein, fats, and carbohydrates it needs to function properly while supporting your weight loss goals.

The Freitas Method encourages nutrient-dense choices. By focusing on the quality of your food, you'll not only achieve a caloric deficit but also ensure that your body is getting the nutrients it needs to stay healthy and energized throughout the process.

Metabolism: Understanding the Process

Your metabolism is the process by which your body converts the food you eat into energy. It's influenced by factors like age, gender, body composition, and activity level.

Resting Metabolic Rate (RMR) refers to the number of calories your body needs at rest to perform basic life-sustaining functions, such as breathing, digestion, and maintaining body temperature. These functions are essential for survival, even when you're not physically active.

A large portion of your daily caloric expenditure is used just to maintain these fundamental functions. For example, even when you're sitting still or sleeping, your body continues to work hard to support processes like circulation, cell repair, and immune function.

One of the most calorically expensive organs in your body is your brain. Although the brain accounts for only about 2% of your total body weight, it uses approximately 20% of your resting metabolic rate. This means that the brain consumes a significant amount of energy even when you're doing nothing but resting.

For example, the brain requires about 300–400 calories per day to function at rest, as it's constantly processing information, regulating body systems, and supporting mental functions like thinking, memory, and concentration. This is why staying mentally engaged can make you feel fatigued — your brain is burning a considerable amount of energy to perform these cognitive tasks.

Understanding your Resting Metabolic Rate (RMR) is key for weight loss, because it shows how much energy your body burns at rest, which contributes to your total daily caloric expenditure. The higher your RMR, the more calories you burn at rest — which is why maintaining muscle mass and staying physically active can help to increase this number.

The Thermic Effect of Food (TEF) refers to the energy your body expends to digest, absorb, and process the food you eat. When you consume food, your body doesn't just "store" calories — it has to work to break down, digest, and metabolize those calories into usable energy. This process requires energy itself.

TEF accounts for about 10% of your total daily caloric expenditure, although this number can vary slightly depending on the composition of the food you eat. For example, protein-rich foods tend to have a higher thermic effect compared to carbohydrates or fats. This is because proteins require more energy for digestion and metabolism due to their complex structure.

Here's a breakdown of how TEF works:

Digestion: After you eat, your stomach begins to break down the food using enzymes and acids. This process requires energy to break down the food into smaller particles that can be absorbed by the intestines.

Absorption: Once the food is broken down into its nutrient components (such as amino acids, glucose, and fatty acids), your intestines absorb these nutrients. Energy is required to transport these nutrients through the intestinal wall into the bloodstream.

Processing: After absorption, the body processes and metabolizes the nutrients. For example, carbohydrates are converted into glucose, fats are stored as fatty acids, and proteins are used for building muscle tissue. All of these steps require energy to facilitate the chemical reactions that turn food into usable fuel.

The amount of energy required for TEF varies depending on the macronutrient composition of the food:

- *Proteins*: Protein has the highest thermic effect, requiring around 20-30% of the energy contained in the protein to be used for digestion and metabolism. This is because proteins are more complex molecules and require more work to break down and process.

- *Carbohydrates*: Carbs have a lower thermic effect, around 5-10% of the energy content of the food. Carbohydrates are simpler molecules compared to proteins and, therefore, require less energy to digest and metabolize.

- *Fats*: Fats have the lowest thermic effect, requiring only 0–3% of their energy content for processing. While fat digestion is slower compared to carbohydrates or protein—due to the need for bile and specific enzymes—it is metabolically efficient, meaning it doesn't require much energy to break down and absorb.

Why TEF Matters ?

The Thermic Effect of Food is an often-overlooked factor in the total calories your body burns each day. While TEF may not be as significant as other factors, such as Resting Metabolic Rate (RMR) or physical activity, it still plays an important role in the overall energy balance. For example, a diet high in protein can slightly boost the number of calories your body burns throughout the day due to the higher thermic effect of protein. This is one reason why high-protein diets are often recommended for people trying to lose weight or maintain muscle mass, as they can help increase energy expenditure.

Additionally, the thermic effect of food can play a role in satiety. Foods with higher TEF (like proteins) may help you feel fuller longer because the body takes more time and energy to process them, leading to greater feelings of fullness and satisfaction.

Incorporating a diet with higher protein content or focusing on nutrient-dense foods can help you slightly increase your total daily energy expenditure, making it a useful strategy for weight loss or maintenance.

Physical Activity: The Energy Expended Through Exercise and Movement

Physical activity plays a critical role in energy expenditure and is one of the most powerful tools for both weight loss and maintaining overall health. This category refers to the energy your body uses when engaging in any form of physical movement, from walking to intense workouts, and it is a major component of your Total Daily Energy Expenditure (TDEE).

When you engage in physical activity, your body requires energy to fuel muscles, sustain heart rate, and support other physiological processes involved in movement. The energy used depends on the intensity and duration of the activity. Even small movements throughout the day, such as walking or fidgeting, contribute to your total energy expenditure, which is why non-exercise activity thermogenesis (NEAT) can also have a significant impact on your metabolism.

How Physical Activity Impacts Metabolism

The Freitas Method recognizes that individuals who engage in regular physical activity generally experience a higher Resting Metabolic Rate (RMR). This is because exercise, particularly strength training and aerobic exercise, can help increase lean muscle mass and improve cardiovascular health. Both of these factors contribute to a more efficient metabolism.

Building Lean Muscle: Muscle tissue is metabolically active, meaning it burns more calories at rest compared to fat tissue. By incorporating strength training into your routine, you can build muscle and increase your basal metabolic rate (BMR), leading to more calories burned throughout the day even when you're not exercising.

Cardiovascular Exercise: Aerobic exercises like running, cycling, or swimming improve cardiovascular health and increase calorie burn during the activity. These exercises also help improve oxygen consumption, which in turn supports more efficient fat burning.

Post-Exercise Energy Expenditure: After intense physical activity, your body continues to burn calories at a higher rate as part of the Excess Post-Exercise Oxygen Consumption (EPOC). This phenomenon, also known as the "afterburn effect," refers to the increased calorie burn that happens after exercise, as your body works to return to its resting state. High-intensity interval training (HIIT) and strength training are particularly effective at triggering EPOC, which makes them powerful tools for weight loss.

The Role of Physical Activity in Weight Loss

For weight loss, caloric expenditure from physical activity is essential, as it helps you create a caloric deficit — the cornerstone of any weight loss program. While diet alone can help you lose weight by restricting calorie intake, adding physical activity to the mix accelerates weight loss and improves long-term results.

Exercise burns calories: The more active you are, the more calories you burn. Regular exercise can help you achieve a greater caloric deficit without the need for extreme dietary restrictions.

Preserving muscle mass: During weight loss, the body not only burns fat but may also break down muscle tissue. Physical activity, particularly resistance training, helps preserve and even build muscle mass, preventing the loss of lean tissue that often accompanies weight loss.

Improving body composition: Physical activity doesn't just affect the number on the scale. It helps you lose fat while maintaining or increasing muscle mass, which can result in a more toned and lean appearance, even if the scale doesn't change drastically.

The Benefits Beyond Weight Loss

While physical activity is an important tool for weight loss, its benefits extend far beyond the scale:

- *Improved cardiovascular health:* Regular physical activity strengthens the heart and blood vessels, reducing the risk of heart disease and improving overall heart function.

- *Increased energy levels:* Consistent exercise boosts energy levels and combats fatigue by improving the efficiency of your cardiovascular and respiratory systems.

- *Mental health:* Exercise has powerful mental health benefits, reducing symptoms of anxiety, depression, and stress. It boosts endorphins, leading to better mood and improved cognitive function.

- *Better sleep:* Regular exercise improves the quality of sleep by helping regulate circadian rhythms and promoting deeper, more restorative sleep.
- *Reduced risk of chronic diseases:* Physical activity helps prevent and manage conditions like Type 2 diabetes, high blood pressure, and obesity, leading to better long-term health outcomes.

Physical Activity in the Freitas Method

The Freitas Method places significant importance on physical activity not only for weight loss but also for enhancing overall metabolic function and well-being. The method encourages individuals to incorporate a balance of strength training, cardio, and flexibility exercises into their routines, depending on personal goals, preferences, and physical limitations.

The daily scoring system tracks the quality and quantity of your physical activity, ensuring that you're consistently challenging yourself to move more. Whether it's a brisk walk, a yoga session, or a vigorous workout, each form of movement contributes to your overall score and supports your progress.

The Importance of Consistency

While creating a caloric deficit is important, consistency is what drives lasting results. The body doesn't respond to short bursts of extreme dieting or exercise. It thrives on sustainable, gradual changes.

The Role of Macronutrients in Weight Loss

Your body requires three main types of macronutrients: carbohydrates, proteins, and fats. Each of these plays a unique role in weight loss and overall health.

- *Carbohydrates* are your body's primary energy source. While some diets restrict carbs, they are an essential nutrient. The key is to focus on complex carbohydrates, such as whole grains, legumes, and vegetables, which provide fiber and steady energy.
- *Proteins* are crucial for muscle repair and growth. When you're in a caloric deficit, maintaining muscle mass is important for keeping your metabolism functioning efficiently. Lean sources of protein, like chicken, fish, tofu, and legumes, should be incorporated into your meals to support your weight loss.

- *Fats* are essential for hormone production and brain function. Healthy fats, such as those found in avocados, nuts, seeds, and olive oil, can help keep you satisfied and provide steady energy throughout the day.

Understanding the balance between these macronutrients is crucial. The Freitas Method helps you align your food choices with your weight loss goals by providing guidelines on how to incorporate these macronutrients in a way that supports both satisfaction and fat loss.

Energy Balance: The Big Picture

While caloric deficit is the foundation of weight loss, energy balance plays a significant role in determining how effectively your body loses or gains weight. Energy balance refers to the relationship between the calories you consume and the calories you burn.

- *Positive energy balance* occurs when you consume more calories than your body needs, leading to weight gain.
- *Negative energy balance* occurs when you consume fewer calories than your body needs, leading to weight loss.
- *Neutral energy balance* occurs when your calorie intake matches your calorie expenditure, which results in weight maintenance.

The Freitas Method encourages you to create a negative energy balance through mindful eating, regular physical activity, and consistent hydration — all while tracking your progress with the scoring system.

The Power of Hydration in Your Weight Loss Journey

When it comes to weight loss, most people immediately think about food and exercise. But there's a silent, often overlooked factor that plays a crucial role in how our body functions and burns fat: hydration.

Why Water Matters? Water is not just a thirst-quencher — it's a key player in nearly every metabolic process in your body. From transporting nutrients and regulating body temperature to flushing out toxins and supporting digestion, water is the fuel behind the scenes.

Even mild dehydration can have noticeable effects: fatigue, poor concentration, headaches, increased cravings, and reduced physical performance. In a weight loss context, these effects can reduce your motivation and hinder your results.

Did you know that water is essential for fat metabolism? The process of lipolysis — the breakdown of fat for energy — requires water to function efficiently. Without enough hydration, your body simply can't burn fat at its full potential.

Studies have also shown that drinking water can temporarily boost your resting metabolic rate. In other words, staying hydrated might help you burn slightly more calories, even while at rest.

Many people confuse thirst with hunger. This can lead to unnecessary snacking or larger meal portions. By staying hydrated throughout the day, you're more likely to be in tune with your actual hunger cues and less prone to overeating.

A simple strategy: when you feel hungry between meals, try drinking a glass of water first and wait 10 minutes. You may realize you were just dehydrated.

How Much Water Do You Need? A common guideline is to aim for 2 to 2.5 liters of plain water per day for most adults. Alternatively, you can follow the rule of 30 to 35 ml per kilogram of body weight. For example, a person weighing 70 kg should drink between 2.1 and 2.45 liters daily.

Hydration should come primarily from water or unsweetened herbal teas. While some hydration does come from food (like fruits and vegetables), it should not replace your daily water intake.

Soft drinks, fruit juices, energy drinks, and alcohol do not count as good hydration sources. In fact, they can dehydrate you further or introduce unnecessary calories and sugars.

Drinking more water is one of the simplest, most effective changes you can make for your health. It doesn't require willpower, special planning, or major lifestyle changes — just awareness and intention.

So next time you're working on your nutrition and physical activity, don't forget your water bottle. Sometimes, the smallest daily habits make the biggest difference.

That's why the Freitas Method places special emphasis on hydration — not just as a supportive tool for weight loss, but as a pillar of overall health. By making water intake a daily habit worth tracking, the method helps you stay consistent, energized, and aligned with your goals. A well-hydrated body functions better, burns fat more efficiently, and feels more balanced — and those are key ingredients for lasting transformation.

7. How the Scoring System Works

The Freitas Method relies on a simple, yet effective, scoring system designed to track your daily behaviors, not just your weight. By assigning points to different actions, you can create clear, actionable goals and consistently evaluate your progress. This system empowers you to understand how small choices add up over time, leading to tangible results.

Daily Scoring Breakdown

The method scores three main areas: nutrition, hydration, and physical activity. Each area is assigned a set number of points, which are totaled to create your daily score. This score will guide you in understanding how well you've adhered to your goals and which areas need improvement.

- *Nutrition:* This section evaluates the quality of your meals, focusing on factors like portion control, balance, and food choices. A well-balanced, nutrient-dense meal earns higher points, while processed or excessive eating will lower your score.

- *Hydration*: Staying properly hydrated is crucial for health and weight loss. This section evaluates your daily water intake, rewarding you for maintaining adequate hydration levels.

- *Physical Activity:* Exercise is a key part of the Freitas Method. Whether it's walking, running, strength training, or other forms of movement, physical activity earns you points based on its intensity and duration. A higher score in this area reflects more engagement in physical activity, which helps support weight loss and overall health.

Daily and weekly Score

At the end of each day, you'll tally the points in each category. Your total score is the sum of your nutrition, hydration, and physical activity points. The score helps you see where you succeeded and where you may need to make adjustments.

For example, you may end the day with a score of +12, with the maximum possible score being +16 — a solid, positive result that shows you made healthy choices across the board. Or, you may get a score of -4, indicating that some areas need attention and improvement. At the end of each week, an average of the points obtained is calculated and then displayed in a bar chart. This allows you to visualize your progress and consistency over the weeks.

Tracking and Feedback

The beauty of the Freitas Method is that feedback is immediate. Each day, you know exactly where you stand. This constant feedback helps you stay motivated and focused, allowing for real-time adjustments and improvements.

The daily score provides an objective way to track progress without obsessing over the scale. While weight loss may fluctuate, your behaviors — and therefore your scores — can consistently improve. Over time, you'll notice patterns, both in your actions and in your results.

Turning Points into Progress

The Freitas Method is designed to show you progress, not perfection. It's about celebrating the small victories every day. A high score isn't a reason to get complacent, but rather an encouragement to keep building on positive habits. A low score isn't failure, but a signal to assess and adjust, giving you the opportunity to bounce back stronger the next day.

Conclusion

As we reach the end of this Part 1, the core message of the Freitas Method should be clear: lasting weight loss and health are built on a foundation of self-awareness, consistency, and sustainable habits. This method is not about quick fixes, extreme restrictions, or relying on willpower alone. Instead, it provides a structured yet flexible framework to help you build positive habits that can be maintained over the long term — whatever your diet or lifestyle.

The Power of Tracking and Scoring

At the heart of the Freitas Method is the daily scoring system, which gives you a tangible way to track your progress. Whether it's the foods you eat, the water you drink, or the physical activity you engage in, assigning points gives you real-time feedback on your choices and helps you stay accountable. By creating a daily score, you take a step back and objectively evaluate your behaviors, allowing you to make adjustments in real time.

This system is designed to empower you to make better decisions, not just in the short term, but as part of a long-term approach to health and weight management. With each passing day, the method helps you establish a routine that becomes second nature, turning healthy choices into lifelong habits.

The Flexibility to Choose Your Path

One of the most powerful aspects of the Freitas Method is its flexibility. The method is not a one-size-fits-all approach; it can be tailored to your specific preferences, lifestyle, and goals. Whether you follow a specific diet like low-carb, vegan, Mediterranean, or intermittent fasting, or simply focus on nutrient-dense foods, the Freitas Method adapts to you.

This adaptability ensures that you can apply the principles of the method no matter your starting point, ensuring that your journey to health is as personalized as it is effective.

Consistency is Key

In a world that often prioritizes instant results, the Freitas Method teaches us that consistency is the real key to success.

The method helps shift your mindset away from seeking quick fixes and toward building habits that you can maintain for life. It's not about perfection — it's about progress. Some days will be better than others, but with the daily and weekly scoring system, you'll have a clear picture of your overall trend. This focus on consistency encourages you to keep moving forward, no matter the obstacles that arise.

Holistic Health Beyond Weight Loss

While the primary goal of the Freitas Method may be weight loss, its principles extend far beyond that. The method emphasizes the importance of hydration, nutrient-dense foods, and regular physical activity, all of which are integral to overall health. It teaches us that weight management is just one piece of the puzzle, and true well-being encompasses physical, mental, and emotional health.

By improving your eating habits, boosting your physical activity, and prioritizing self-care, the Freitas Method guides you toward a more holistic approach to health. The daily scoring system becomes a tool to not only track your weight but also monitor your mental and physical well-being.

The Journey Ahead

This book has provided you with the knowledge, tools, and framework to begin your journey toward lasting health and weight loss. However, the real work begins now. Every day is an opportunity to make choices that align with your goals. Whether you're just starting your journey or you're already well on your way, the Freitas Method provides the structure you need to stay consistent and accountable, no matter where you are.

Remember, weight loss and health are not just about achieving a number on the scale; they are about creating habits that help you live a fuller, healthier life. The Freitas Method offers a roadmap that empowers you to embrace a balanced approach, supporting your goals without resorting to extreme measures or temporary fixes.

Final Thoughts

Achieving your health goals requires more than just following a diet — it requires commitment, patience, and a willingness to make lasting changes.

By embracing the principles of the Freitas Method, you are choosing a path of sustainable, long-term health. The method is designed to help you build a foundation of healthy habits, which can improve your life far beyond weight loss.

You now have the tools to make better choices, stay consistent, and build a healthy, active life. The journey may be challenging at times, but it is one worth taking. And remember, you are not alone — by following the Freitas Method, you are joining a community of people committed to improving their lives, one day at a time.

The path to health and well-being is in your hands.

Now, it's time to begin.

In **Part 2** of this book, we will dive into the practical application of the Freitas Method, where you can implement the concepts discussed here into your everyday routine. You will have access to tools and resources to guide you through the process, helping you to stay on track and achieve your personal health goals.

Part Two

Instrutions

Each day, you will assign a score—based on the provided criteria—for hydration, for each of the five daily meals, and for physical activity. Then, you'll add up the points and record the total at the end of the day, as shown in the example below.

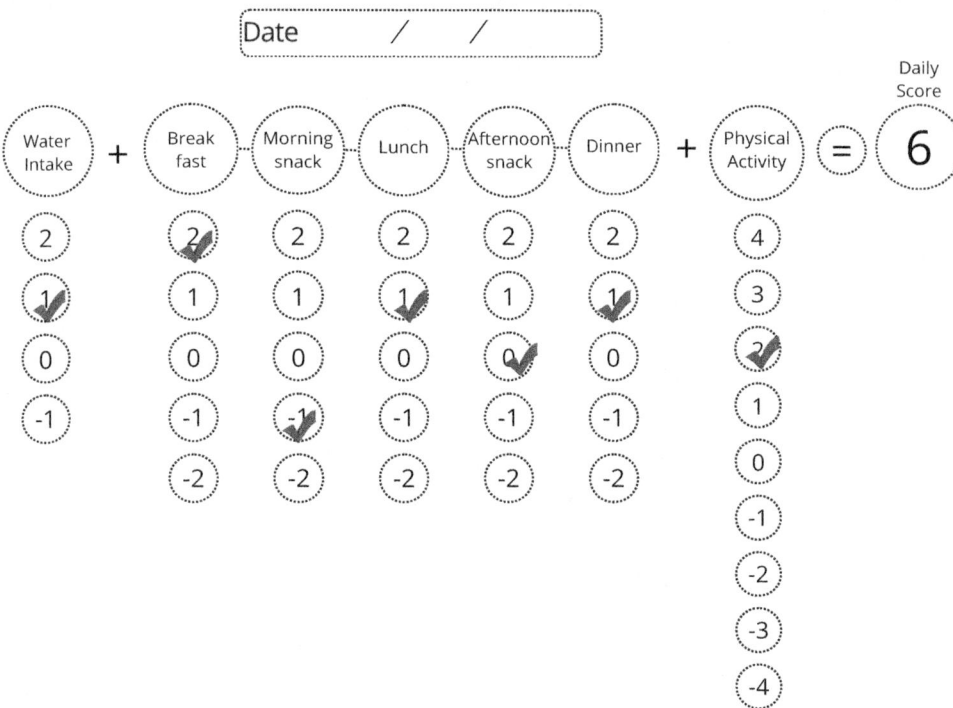

While the scoring system in this book provides general reference values, it's important to remember that every individual is different. Factors such as weight, fitness level, age, metabolism, and specific health goals can influence your needs and capacities. The Freitas Method is designed to be flexible — you are encouraged to adapt the criteria to better reflect your personal context. What matters most is consistency and honesty in your self-assessment. Adjusting the system to suit your reality doesn't weaken it — it makes it more sustainable and effective for you.

Freitas Method – Hydration Scoring Scale		
Water Intake (per day)*	**Score**	**Interpretation**
≥ 2.0 to 2.5 liters	2	Optimal hydration
1.5 to 2 liters	1	Acceptable, but below the optimal range
1.0 to 1.5 liters	0	Insufficient hydration
0 to 1 liters	-1	Poor hydration

* This should be water consumed in the form of water or unsweetened herbal tea. The water content in food or other beverages should not be counted. You can also choose to use the formula of 30 to 35 ml per kilogram of body weight. The key idea to remember is: the larger the body, the more water it needs.

Certain conditions or lifestyle factors can increase your daily hydration requirements:
- Intense physical activity
- Hot or dry climates
- High-protein or high-fiber diets
- Illness (e.g., fever, vomiting, diarrhea)
- Certain medications

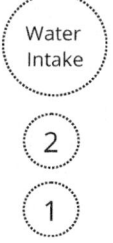

Freitas Method – Food Scoring Scale

Meal Quality	Score	Explanation
Meal does not exist	1	Fewer calories consumed; aligns with intermittent fasting principles, but not a suggestion to skip all meals.
Healthy and in reasonable quantity	2	A balanced, healthy meal in an appropriate portion size.
Healthy but in excess	1	A healthy meal but eaten in excess.
Neutral meal	0	A meal that is not particularly healthy or unhealthy.
Unhealthy meal	-1	A meal that is unhealthy but not excessively large.
Unhealthy and in excess	-2	An unhealthy meal consumed in large quantities.
Includes ice cream, cakes, soft drinks, or French fries	-1 per item	Deduction of 1 point for each of these items included (e.g., 2 soft drinks = -2 points).

Break fast	Morning snack	Lunch	Afternoon snack	Dinner
2	2	2	2	2
1	1	1	1	1
0	0	0	0	0
-1	-1	-1	-1	-1
-2	-2	-2	-2	-2

Freitas Method – Physical Activity Scoring Scale		
Activity Type	**Score**	**Explanation**
Walking – 20 minutes	1	Light to moderate activity, encourages regular movement throughout the day.
Running – 10 minutes	1	Higher intensity, burns more calories in less time.
Other intense activities – 10 minutes	1	Includes cycling, swimming, gym workouts, HIIT, etc.
Sitting – every 2 hours continuously	-1	Penalty for prolonged sedentary time without active breaks.

Rules for Daily Scoring:

Physical Activity

- Combine time from multiple activities throughout the day. (e.g., 40 minutes walking + 20 minutes gym = +4 points)
- Deduct 1 point for every 2 hours of uninterrupted sitting (e.g., 6 hours seated = -3 points)
- The final score for physical activity can be positive or negative depending on the balance between movement and sedentary behavior.

4
3
2
1
0
-1
-2
-3
-4

Freitas Method – Daily/Weekly Score Classification

Score Range	Classification	Implications for Weight & Health
+13 to +16	Excellent	Strong weight loss potential. Consistent healthy habits and high activity.
+9 to +12.9	Very Good	Moderate to steady weight loss. Good balance of diet and activity.
+5 to +8.9	Good	Slight weight loss or maintenance. Mostly healthy choices.
+1 to +4.9	Neutral	Likely weight maintenance. Inconsistent effort or light improvement.
0 to -4.9	Poor	Risk of weight gain. Frequent unhealthy choices or lack of activity.
-5 to -8.9	Very Poor	Active weight gain. Unbalanced eating, low movement, high sedentary time.
-9 to -15	Critical	Significant health risk. Persistent negative behaviors, low awareness.

Part Three

In the following pages, we'll move into Part 3 of the book — your personal tracking zone, where real transformation begins. Each page represents one full day of your journey, providing space for you to log your hydration, meals, physical activity, and your total daily score. The scoring criteria are included on each page for easy reference, especially in the beginning. Over time, as your understanding deepens and healthy habits become second nature, you'll likely find yourself needing to consult them less and less — a sign that your mindset is shifting and your lifestyle is changing.

At the end of the book, you'll find weekly summary chart. These allow you to collect your daily scores and visualize your progress in a simple bar graph format. This weekly reflection is more than just numbers — it's a mirror of your consistency, your effort, and your growth. Watching your progress build over time can be incredibly motivating. It turns your journey into something you can see, track, and feel proud of.

And remember: not every day will be perfect — and that's okay. The goal isn't perfection, it's progress. A low score isn't failure, it's feedback. It's a chance to reflect, adjust, and come back stronger tomorrow. The Freitas Method is about long-term success, built one day at a time, through small, sustainable actions that compound into lasting change. Stay committed, stay patient, and above all, stay kind to yourself. You're building more than a score — you're building a healthier, more empowered version of yourself.

Before you begin, I want to take a moment to thank you — not just for reading this book, but for choosing to invest in yourself. The fact that you're here, ready to take responsibility and create positive change, already puts you ahead. Every page you fill is a small act of courage, a declaration that you are committed to your health, your well-being, and your future.

Remember, transformation doesn't happen overnight — it happens in the quiet consistency of daily effort. Some days will be easier than others, but every step forward counts.

I created this method not as a set of rules, but as a companion for your journey — a tool to help you stay focused, motivated, and accountable. You are not alone in this process, and I truly believe that if you show up for yourself every day with honesty and intention, lasting results will follow.

With gratitude,
António Freitas

Date　　　/　　/　　　　Week 1

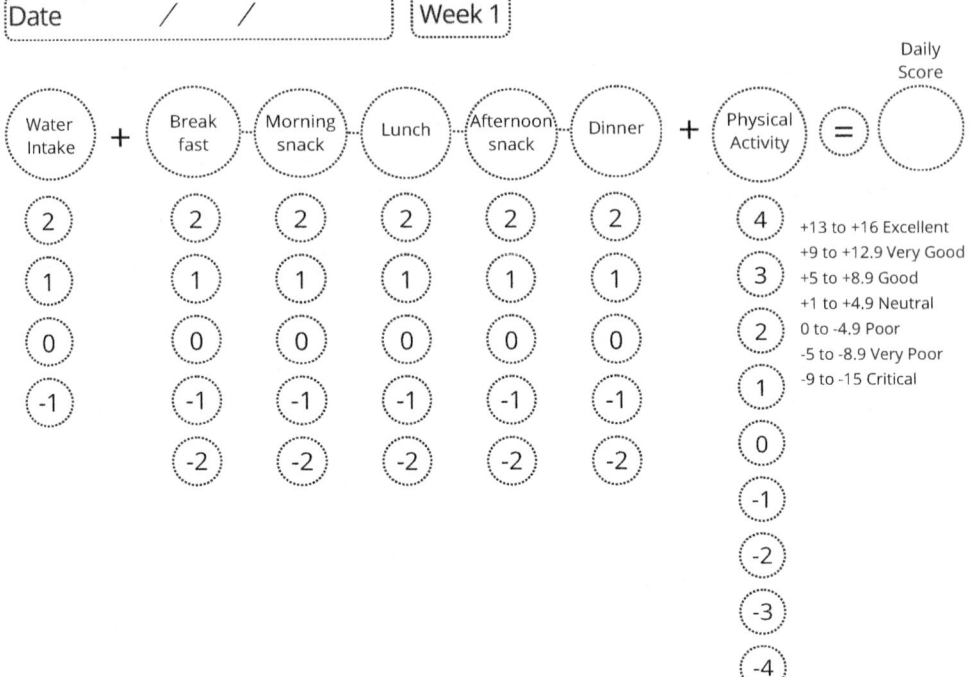

| Water Intake | + | Break fast | Morning snack | Lunch | Afternoon snack | Dinner | + | Physical Activity | = | Daily Score |

+13 to +16 Excellent
+9 to +12.9 Very Good
+5 to +8.9 Good
+1 to +4.9 Neutral
0 to -4.9 Poor
-5 to -8.9 Very Poor
-9 to -15 Critical

Hydration Scoring Scale

Water Intake (per day)*	Score
≥ 2.0 to 2.5 liters	2
1.5 to 2 liters	1
1 to 1.5 liters	0
0 to 1 liters	-1

Food Scoring Scale

Meal Quality	Score
Meal does not exist	1
Healthy and in reasonable quantity	2
Healthy but in excess	1
Neutral meal	0
Unhealthy meal	-1
Unhealthy and in excess	-2
Includes ice cream, cakes, soft drinks, or French fries	-1 per item

Physical Activity Scoring Scale

Activity Type	Score
Walking – 15 minutes	1
Running – 10 minutes	1
Other intense activities – 10 minutes	1
Sitting – every 2 hours continuously	-1

Daily Score

Water Intake **+** Break fast — Morning snack — Lunch — Afternoon snack — Dinner **+** Physical Activity **=** ( )

Water Intake	Break fast	Morning snack	Lunch	Afternoon snack	Dinner	Physical Activity
2	2	2	2	2	2	4
1	1	1	1	1	1	3
0	0	0	0	0	0	2
-1	-1	-1	-1	-1	-1	1
	-2	-2	-2	-2	-2	0
						-1
						-2
						-3
						-4

+13 to +16 Excellent
+9 to +12.9 Very Good
+5 to +8.9 Good
+1 to +4.9 Neutral
0 to -4.9 Poor
-5 to -8.9 Very Poor
-9 to -15 Critical

Hydration Scoring Scale

Water Intake (per day)*	Score
≥ 2.0 to 2.5 liters	2
1.5 to 2 liters	1
1 to 1.5 liters	0
0 to 1 liters	-1

Food Scoring Scale

Meal Quality	Score
Meal does not exist	1
Healthy and in reasonable quantity	2
Healthy but in excess	1
Neutral meal	0
Unhealthy meal	-1
Unhealthy and in excess	-2
Includes ice cream, cakes, soft drinks, or French fries	-1 per item

Physical Activity Scoring Scale

Activity Type	Score
Walking – 15 minutes	1
Running – 10 minutes	1
Other intense activities – 10 minutes	1
Sitting – every 2 hours continuously	-1

Date	/ /	Week 1

Daily Score

(Water Intake) + (Break fast) (Morning snack) (Lunch) (Afternoon snack) (Dinner) + (Physical Activity) (=) ( )

Water Intake	Break fast	Morning snack	Lunch	Afternoon snack	Dinner	Physical Activity
2	2	2	2	2	2	4
1	1	1	1	1	1	3
0	0	0	0	0	0	2
-1	-1	-1	-1	-1	-1	1
	-2	-2	-2	-2	-2	0
						-1
						-2
						-3
						-4

+13 to +16 Excellent
+9 to +12.9 Very Good
+5 to +8.9 Good
+1 to +4.9 Neutral
0 to -4.9 Poor
-5 to -8.9 Very Poor
-9 to -15 Critical

Hydration Scoring Scale

Water Intake (per day)*	Score
≥ 2.0 to 2.5 liters	2
1.5 to 2 liters	1
1 to 1.5 liters	0
0 to 1 liters	-1

Food Scoring Scale

Meal Quality	Score
Meal does not exist	1
Healthy and in reasonable quantity	2
Healthy but in excess	1
Neutral meal	0
Unhealthy meal	-1
Unhealthy and in excess	-2
Includes ice cream, cakes, soft drinks, or French fries	-1 per item

Physical Activity Scoring Scale

Activity Type	Score
Walking – 15 minutes	1
Running – 10 minutes	1
Other intense activities – 10 minutes	1
Sitting – every 2 hours continuously	-1

Date	/	/	Week 1

Daily
Score

Water Intake $+$ Break fast + Morning snack + Lunch + Afternoon snack + Dinner $+$ Physical Activity $=$ ( )

Water Intake	Break fast	Morning snack	Lunch	Afternoon snack	Dinner	Physical Activity
2	2	2	2	2	2	4
1	1	1	1	1	1	3
0	0	0	0	0	0	2
-1	-1	-1	-1	-1	-1	1
	-2	-2	-2	-2	-2	0
						-1
						-2
						-3
						-4

+13 to +16 Excellent
+9 to +12.9 Very Good
+5 to +8.9 Good
+1 to +4.9 Neutral
0 to -4.9 Poor
-5 to -8.9 Very Poor
-9 to -15 Critical

Hydration Scoring Scale

Water Intake (per day)*	Score
≥ 2.0 to 2.5 liters	2
1.5 to 2 liters	1
1 to 1.5 liters	0
0 to 1 liters	-1

Food Scoring Scale

Meal Quality	Score
Meal does not exist	1
Healthy and in reasonable quantity	2
Healthy but in excess	1
Neutral meal	0
Unhealthy meal	-1
Unhealthy and in excess	-2
Includes ice cream, cakes, soft drinks, or French fries	-1 per item

Physical Activity Scoring Scale

Activity Type	Score
Walking – 15 minutes	1
Running – 10 minutes	1
Other intense activities – 10 minutes	1
Sitting – every 2 hours continuously	-1

Date	/	/		Week 1

Daily Score

(Water Intake) + (Breakfast) (Morning snack) (Lunch) (Afternoon snack) (Dinner) + (Physical Activity) = ( )

Water Intake	Breakfast	Morning snack	Lunch	Afternoon snack	Dinner	Physical Activity	
2	2	2	2	2	2	4	+13 to +16 Excellent
1	1	1	1	1	1	3	+9 to +12.9 Very Good
0	0	0	0	0	0	2	+5 to +8.9 Good
-1	-1	-1	-1	-1	-1	1	+1 to +4.9 Neutral
	-2	-2	-2	-2	-2	0	0 to -4.9 Poor
						-1	-5 to -8.9 Very Poor
						-2	-9 to -15 Critical
						-3	
						-4	

Hydration Scoring Scale

Water Intake (per day)*	Score
≥ 2.0 to 2.5 liters	2
1.5 to 2 liters	1
1 to 1.5 liters	0
0 to 1 liters	-1

Food Scoring Scale

Meal Quality	Score
Meal does not exist	1
Healthy and in reasonable quantity	2
Healthy but in excess	1
Neutral meal	0
Unhealthy meal	-1
Unhealthy and in excess	-2
Includes ice cream, cakes, soft drinks, or French fries	-1 per item

Physical Activity Scoring Scale

Activity Type	Score
Walking – 15 minutes	1
Running – 10 minutes	1
Other intense activities – 10 minutes	1
Sitting – every 2 hours continuously	-1

Date / /	Week 1

Daily Score

(Water Intake) + (Break fast) (Morning snack) (Lunch) (Afternoon snack) (Dinner) + (Physical Activity) = ( )

Water Intake: 2, 1, 0, -1

Break fast: 2, 1, 0, -1, -2

Morning snack: 2, 1, 0, -1, -2

Lunch: 2, 1, 0, -1, -2

Afternoon snack: 2, 1, 0, -1, -2

Dinner: 2, 1, 0, -1, -2

Physical Activity: 4, 3, 2, 1, 0, -1, -2, -3, -4

+13 to +16 Excellent
+9 to +12.9 Very Good
+5 to +8.9 Good
+1 to +4.9 Neutral
0 to -4.9 Poor
-5 to -8.9 Very Poor
-9 to -15 Critical

Hydration Scoring Scale

Water Intake (per day)*	Score
≥ 2.0 to 2.5 liters	2
1.5 to 2 liters	1
1 to 1.5 liters	0
0 to 1 liters	-1

Food Scoring Scale

Meal Quality	Score
Meal does not exist	1
Healthy and in reasonable quantity	2
Healthy but in excess	1
Neutral meal	0
Unhealthy meal	-1
Unhealthy and in excess	-2
Includes ice cream, cakes, soft drinks, or French fries	-1 per item

Physical Activity Scoring Scale

Activity Type	Score
Walking – 15 minutes	1
Running – 10 minutes	1
Other intense activities – 10 minutes	1
Sitting – every 2 hours continuously	-1

Daily Score

(Water Intake) + (Break fast) (Morning snack) (Lunch) (Afternoon snack) (Dinner) + (Physical Activity) = (   )

Water Intake		Break fast	Morning snack	Lunch	Afternoon snack	Dinner		Physical Activity	
2		2	2	2	2	2		4	+13 to +16 Excellent
1		1	1	1	1	1		3	+9 to +12.9 Very Good
0		0	0	0	0	0		2	+5 to +8.9 Good
-1		-1	-1	-1	-1	-1		1	+1 to +4.9 Neutral
		-2	-2	-2	-2	-2		0	0 to -4.9 Poor
								-1	-5 to -8.9 Very Poor
								-2	-9 to -15 Critical
								-3	
								-4	

End of Week 1 – Weekly Summary

At the end of the first week, you should add up all your daily scores and divide the total by 7. This will give you your weekly average, which may be a decimal number.

Record this result in the weekly progress chart located at the end of the book.

Tracking your weekly average will help you visualize your consistency, spot trends, and stay motivated as you move forward on your journey.

Keep going — every step counts!

Date ___ / ___ / ___   Week 2

Daily Score

| Water Intake | + | Break fast | Morning snack | Lunch | Afternoon snack | Dinner | + | Physical Activity | = | ( ) |

Water Intake:
2
1
0
-1

Breakfast:
2
1
0
-1
-2

Morning snack:
2
1
0
-1
-2

Lunch:
2
1
0
-1
-2

Afternoon snack:
2
1
0
-1
-2

Dinner:
2
1
0
-1
-2

Physical Activity:
4
3
2
1
0
-1
-2
-3
-4

+13 to +16 Excellent
+9 to +12.9 Very Good
+5 to +8.9 Good
+1 to +4.9 Neutral
0 to -4.9 Poor
-5 to -8.9 Very Poor
-9 to -15 Critical

Hydration Scoring Scale

Water Intake (per day)*	Score
≥ 2.0 to 2.5 liters	2
1.5 to 2 liters	1
1 to 1.5 liters	0
0 to 1 liters	-1

Food Scoring Scale

Meal Quality	Score
Meal does not exist	1
Healthy and in reasonable quantity	2
Healthy but in excess	1
Neutral meal	0
Unhealthy meal	-1
Unhealthy and in excess	-2
Includes ice cream, cakes, soft drinks, or French fries	-1 per item

Physical Activity Scoring Scale

Activity Type	Score
Walking – 15 minutes	1
Running – 10 minutes	1
Other intense activities – 10 minutes	1
Sitting – every 2 hours continuously	-1

Daily Score

(Water Intake) + (Break fast) (Morning snack) (Lunch) (Afternoon snack) (Dinner) + (Physical Activity) = ( )

Water Intake	Break fast	Morning snack	Lunch	Afternoon snack	Dinner	Physical Activity
2	2	2	2	2	2	4
1	1	1	1	1	1	3
0	0	0	0	0	0	2
-1	-1	-1	-1	-1	-1	1
	-2	-2	-2	-2	-2	0
						-1
						-2
						-3
						-4

+13 to +16 Excellent
+9 to +12.9 Very Good
+5 to +8.9 Good
+1 to +4.9 Neutral
0 to -4.9 Poor
-5 to -8.9 Very Poor
-9 to -15 Critical

Hydration Scoring Scale

Water Intake (per day)*	Score
≥ 2.0 to 2.5 liters	2
1.5 to 2 liters	1
1 to 1.5 liters	0
0 to 1 liters	-1

Food Scoring Scale

Meal Quality	Score
Meal does not exist	1
Healthy and in reasonable quantity	2
Healthy but in excess	1
Neutral meal	0
Unhealthy meal	-1
Unhealthy and in excess	-2
Includes ice cream, cakes, soft drinks, or French fries	-1 per item

Physical Activity Scoring Scale

Activity Type	Score
Walking – 15 minutes	1
Running – 10 minutes	1
Other intense activities – 10 minutes	1
Sitting – every 2 hours continuously	-1

Daily Score

Water Intake + Breakfast · Morning snack · Lunch · Afternoon snack · Dinner + Physical Activity = ( )

Water Intake: 2, 1, 0, -1

Breakfast: 2, 1, 0, -1, -2

Morning snack: 2, 1, 0, -1, -2

Lunch: 2, 1, 0, -1, -2

Afternoon snack: 2, 1, 0, -1, -2

Dinner: 2, 1, 0, -1, -2

Physical Activity: 4, 3, 2, 1, 0, -1, -2, -3, -4

+13 to +16 Excellent
+9 to +12.9 Very Good
+5 to +8.9 Good
+1 to +4.9 Neutral
0 to -4.9 Poor
-5 to -8.9 Very Poor
-9 to -15 Critical

Hydration Scoring Scale

Water Intake (per day)*	Score
≥ 2.0 to 2.5 liters	2
1.5 to 2 liters	1
1 to 1.5 liters	0
0 to 1 liters	-1

Food Scoring Scale

Meal Quality	Score
Meal does not exist	1
Healthy and in reasonable quantity	2
Healthy but in excess	1
Neutral meal	0
Unhealthy meal	-1
Unhealthy and in excess	-2
Includes ice cream, cakes, soft drinks, or French fries	-1 per item

Physical Activity Scoring Scale

Activity Type	Score
Walking – 15 minutes	1
Running – 10 minutes	1
Other intense activities – 10 minutes	1
Sitting – every 2 hours continuously	-1

Date	/	/		Week 2

Daily Score

(Water Intake) + (Break fast) (Morning snack) (Lunch) (Afternoon snack) (Dinner) + (Physical Activity) = ( )

Water Intake	Break fast	Morning snack	Lunch	Afternoon snack	Dinner		Physical Activity	
2	2	2	2	2	2		4	+13 to +16 Excellent
1	1	1	1	1	1		3	+9 to +12.9 Very Good
0	0	0	0	0	0			+5 to +8.9 Good
-1	-1	-1	-1	-1	-1		2	+1 to +4.9 Neutral
	-2	-2	-2	-2	-2		1	0 to -4.9 Poor
							0	-5 to -8.9 Very Poor
							-1	-9 to -15 Critical
							-2	
							-3	
							-4	

Hydration Scoring Scale

Water Intake (per day)*	Score
≥ 2.0 to 2.5 liters	2
1.5 to 2 liters	1
1 to 1.5 liters	0
0 to 1 liters	-1

Food Scoring Scale

Meal Quality	Score
Meal does not exist	1
Healthy and in reasonable quantity	2
Healthy but in excess	1
Neutral meal	0
Unhealthy meal	-1
Unhealthy and in excess	-2
Includes ice cream, cakes, soft drinks, or French fries	-1 per item

Physical Activity Scoring Scale

Activity Type	Score
Walking – 15 minutes	1
Running – 10 minutes	1
Other intense activities – 10 minutes	1
Sitting – every 2 hours continuously	-1

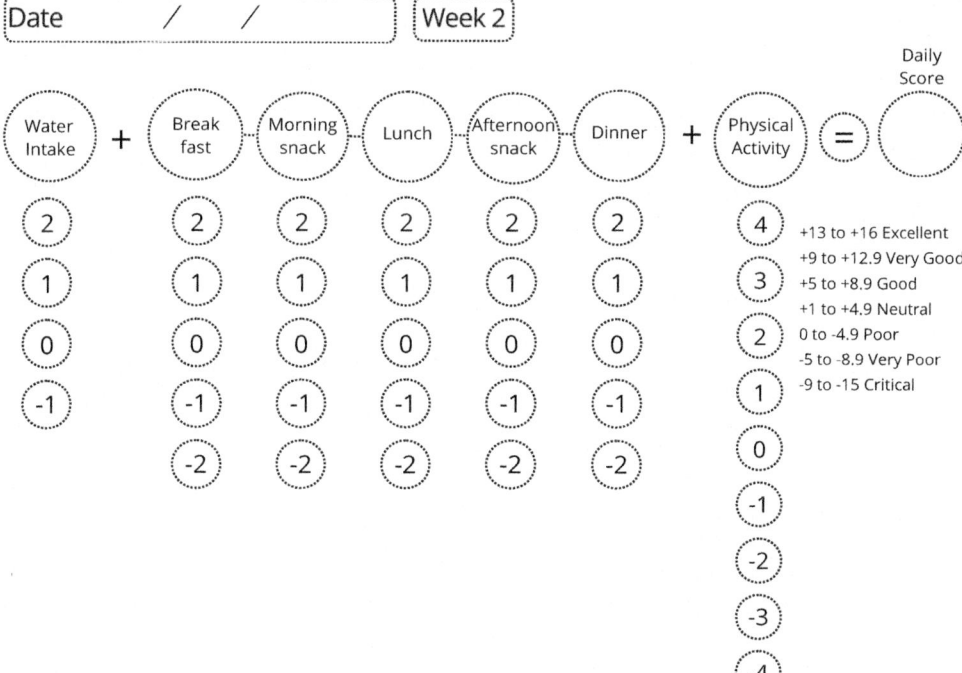

| Date   /   / | Week 2 |

Daily Score

Water Intake + Break fast Morning snack Lunch Afternoon snack Dinner + Physical Activity = ◯

Water Intake: 2, 1, 0, -1

Break fast: 2, 1, 0, -1, -2

Morning snack: 2, 1, 0, -1, -2

Lunch: 2, 1, 0, -1, -2

Afternoon snack: 2, 1, 0, -1, -2

Dinner: 2, 1, 0, -1, -2

Physical Activity: 4, 3, 2, 1, 0, -1, -2, -3, -4

+13 to +16 Excellent
+9 to +12.9 Very Good
+5 to +8.9 Good
+1 to +4.9 Neutral
0 to -4.9 Poor
-5 to -8.9 Very Poor
-9 to -15 Critical

Hydration Scoring Scale

Water Intake (per day)*	Score
≥ 2.0 to 2.5 liters	2
1.5 to 2 liters	1
1 to 1.5 liters	0
0 to 1 liters	-1

Food Scoring Scale

Meal Quality	Score
Meal does not exist	1
Healthy and in reasonable quantity	2
Healthy but in excess	1
Neutral meal	0
Unhealthy meal	-1
Unhealthy and in excess	-2
Includes ice cream, cakes, soft drinks, or French fries	-1 per item

Physical Activity Scoring Scale

Activity Type	Score
Walking – 15 minutes	1
Running – 10 minutes	1
Other intense activities – 10 minutes	1
Sitting – every 2 hours continuously	-1

Date ____ / ____ / ____   Week 2

Daily Score

(Water Intake) + (Break fast) (Morning snack) (Lunch) (Afternoon snack) (Dinner) + (Physical Activity) = ( )

Water Intake	Break fast	Morning snack	Lunch	Afternoon snack	Dinner	Physical Activity	
2	2	2	2	2	2	4	+13 to +16 Excellent
1	1	1	1	1	1	3	+9 to +12.9 Very Good
0	0	0	0	0	0	2	+5 to +8.9 Good
-1	-1	-1	-1	-1	-1	1	+1 to +4.9 Neutral
	-2	-2	-2	-2	-2	0	0 to -4.9 Poor
						-1	-5 to -8.9 Very Poor
						-2	-9 to -15 Critical
						-3	
						-4	

Hydration Scoring Scale

Water Intake (per day)*	Score
≥ 2.0 to 2.5 liters	2
1.5 to 2 liters	1
1 to 1.5 liters	0
0 to 1 liters	-1

Food Scoring Scale

Meal Quality	Score
Meal does not exist	1
Healthy and in reasonable quantity	2
Healthy but in excess	1
Neutral meal	0
Unhealthy meal	-1
Unhealthy and in excess	-2
Includes ice cream, cakes, soft drinks, or French fries	-1 per item

Physical Activity Scoring Scale

Activity Type	Score
Walking – 15 minutes	1
Running – 10 minutes	1
Other intense activities – 10 minutes	1
Sitting – every 2 hours continuously	-1

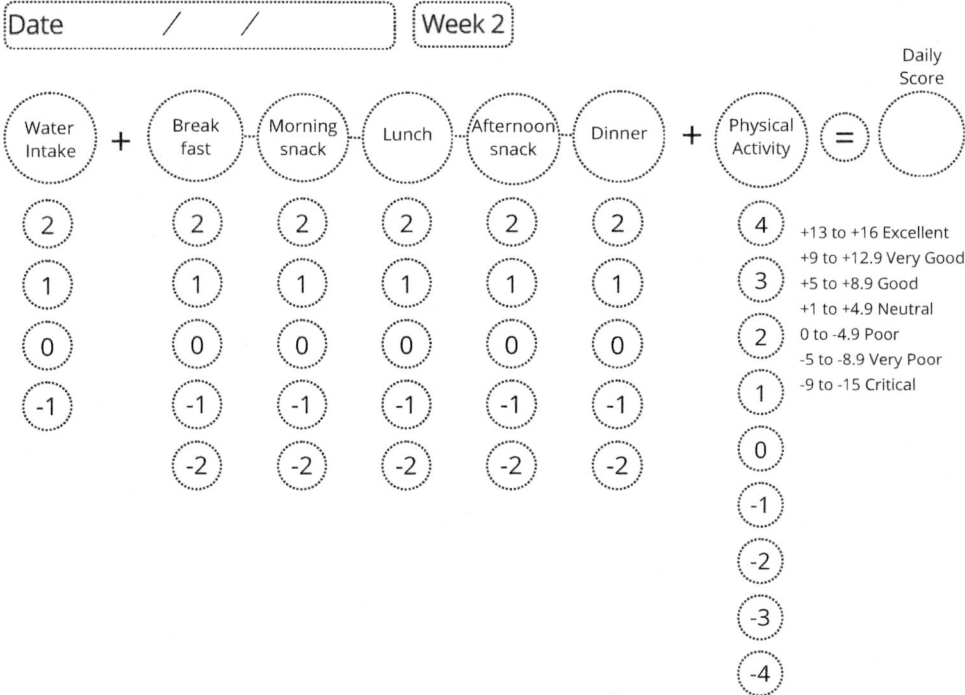

Date ___ / ___ / ___   Week 2

| Water Intake | + | Break fast | Morning snack | Lunch | Afternoon snack | Dinner | + | Physical Activity | = | Daily Score |

+13 to +16 Excellent
+9 to +12.9 Very Good
+5 to +8.9 Good
+1 to +4.9 Neutral
0 to -4.9 Poor
-5 to -8.9 Very Poor
-9 to -15 Critical

End of Week 2 – Weekly Summary

Two weeks down, and every choice you've made is building the foundation for lasting change. Stay focused — your progress is already taking shape!

Daily Score

(Water Intake) + (Break fast) (Morning snack) (Lunch) (Afternoon snack) (Dinner) + (Physical Activity) (=) ( )

Water Intake	Break fast	Morning snack	Lunch	Afternoon snack	Dinner	Physical Activity
2	2	2	2	2	2	4
1	1	1	1	1	1	3
0	0	0	0	0	0	2
-1	-1	-1	-1	-1	-1	1
	-2	-2	-2	-2	-2	0
						-1
						-2
						-3
						-4

+13 to +16 Excellent
+9 to +12.9 Very Good
+5 to +8.9 Good
+1 to +4.9 Neutral
0 to -4.9 Poor
-5 to -8.9 Very Poor
-9 to -15 Critical

Hydration Scoring Scale

Water Intake (per day)*	Score
≥ 2.0 to 2.5 liters	2
1.5 to 2 liters	1
1 to 1.5 liters	0
0 to 1 liters	-1

Food Scoring Scale

Meal Quality	Score
Meal does not exist	1
Healthy and in reasonable quantity	2
Healthy but in excess	1
Neutral meal	0
Unhealthy meal	-1
Unhealthy and in excess	-2
Includes ice cream, cakes, soft drinks, or French fries	-1 per item

Physical Activity Scoring Scale

Activity Type	Score
Walking – 15 minutes	1
Running – 10 minutes	1
Other intense activities – 10 minutes	1
Sitting – every 2 hours continuously	-1

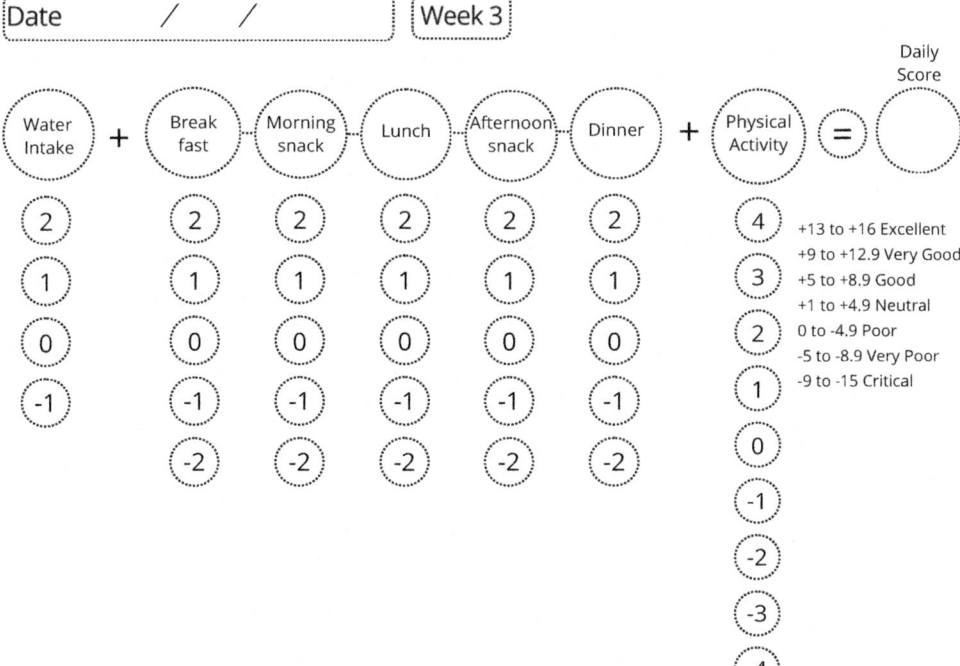

Date ___ / ___ / ___   Week 3

Water Intake + Breakfast + Morning snack + Lunch + Afternoon snack + Dinner + Physical Activity = Daily Score

Water Intake: 2, 1, 0, -1

Breakfast: 2, 1, 0, -1, -2

Morning snack: 2, 1, 0, -1, -2

Lunch: 2, 1, 0, -1, -2

Afternoon snack: 2, 1, 0, -1, -2

Dinner: 2, 1, 0, -1, -2

Physical Activity: 4, 3, 2, 1, 0, -1, -2, -3, -4

+13 to +16 Excellent
+9 to +12.9 Very Good
+5 to +8.9 Good
+1 to +4.9 Neutral
0 to -4.9 Poor
-5 to -8.9 Very Poor
-9 to -15 Critical

Hydration Scoring Scale

Water Intake (per day)*	Score
≥ 2.0 to 2.5 liters	2
1.5 to 2 liters	1
1 to 1.5 liters	0
0 to 1 liters	-1

Food Scoring Scale

Meal Quality	Score
Meal does not exist	1
Healthy and in reasonable quantity	2
Healthy but in excess	1
Neutral meal	0
Unhealthy meal	-1
Unhealthy and in excess	-2
Includes ice cream, cakes, soft drinks, or French fries	-1 per item

Physical Activity Scoring Scale

Activity Type	Score
Walking – 15 minutes	1
Running – 10 minutes	1
Other intense activities – 10 minutes	1
Sitting – every 2 hours continuously	-1

Date ____ / ____ / ____   Week 3

Daily Score

(Water Intake) + (Break fast) (Morning snack) (Lunch) (Afternoon snack) (Dinner) + (Physical Activity) = ( )

Water Intake	Breakfast	Morning snack	Lunch	Afternoon snack	Dinner	Physical Activity
2	2	2	2	2	2	4
1	1	1	1	1	1	3
0	0	0	0	0	0	2
-1	-1	-1	-1	-1	-1	1
	-2	-2	-2	-2	-2	0
						-1
						-2
						-3
						-4

+13 to +16 Excellent
+9 to +12.9 Very Good
+5 to +8.9 Good
+1 to +4.9 Neutral
0 to -4.9 Poor
-5 to -8.9 Very Poor
-9 to -15 Critical

Hydration Scoring Scale

Water Intake (per day)*	Score
≥ 2.0 to 2.5 liters	2
1.5 to 2 liters	1
1 to 1.5 liters	0
0 to 1 liters	-1

Food Scoring Scale

Meal Quality	Score
Meal does not exist	1
Healthy and in reasonable quantity	2
Healthy but in excess	1
Neutral meal	0
Unhealthy meal	-1
Unhealthy and in excess	-2
Includes ice cream, cakes, soft drinks, or French fries	-1 per item

Physical Activity Scoring Scale

Activity Type	Score
Walking – 15 minutes	1
Running – 10 minutes	1
Other intense activities – 10 minutes	1
Sitting – every 2 hours continuously	-1

Daily Score

(Water Intake) + (Break fast) (Morning snack) (Lunch) (Afternoon snack) (Dinner) + (Physical Activity) = ( )

Water Intake	Break fast	Morning snack	Lunch	Afternoon snack	Dinner	Physical Activity	
2	2	2	2	2	2	4	+13 to +16 Excellent
1	1	1	1	1	1	3	+9 to +12.9 Very Good
0	0	0	0	0	0	2	+5 to +8.9 Good
-1	-1	-1	-1	-1	-1	1	+1 to +4.9 Neutral
	-2	-2	-2	-2	-2	0	0 to -4.9 Poor
						-1	-5 to -8.9 Very Poor
						-2	-9 to -15 Critical
						-3	
						-4	

Hydration Scoring Scale

Water Intake (per day)*	Score
≥ 2.0 to 2.5 liters	2
1.5 to 2 liters	1
1 to 1.5 liters	0
0 to 1 liters	-1

Food Scoring Scale

Meal Quality	Score
Meal does not exist	1
Healthy and in reasonable quantity	2
Healthy but in excess	1
Neutral meal	0
Unhealthy meal	-1
Unhealthy and in excess	-2
Includes ice cream, cakes, soft drinks, or French fries	-1 per item

Physical Activity Scoring Scale

Activity Type	Score
Walking – 15 minutes	1
Running – 10 minutes	1
Other intense activities – 10 minutes	1
Sitting – every 2 hours continuously	-1

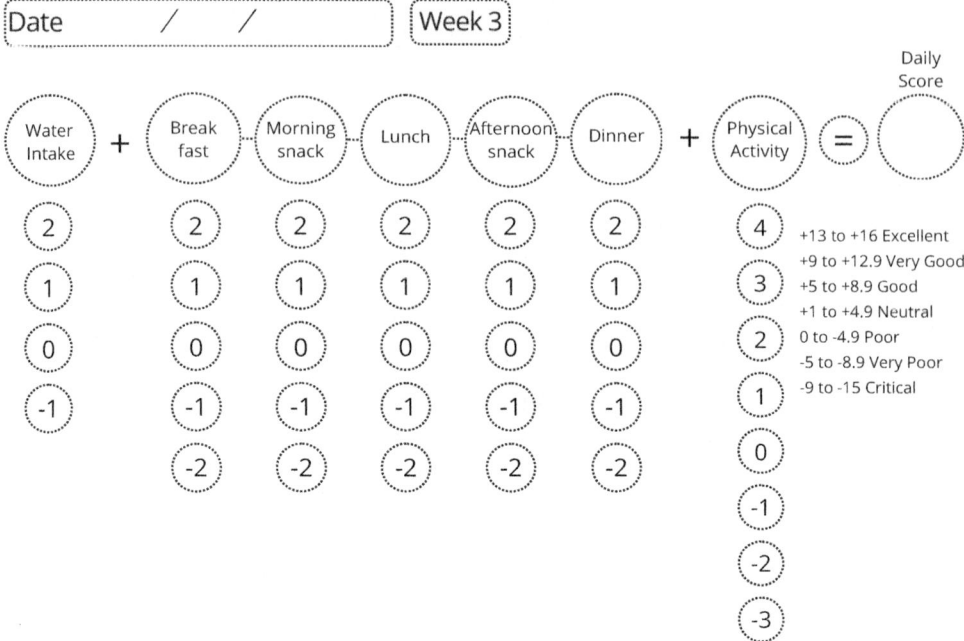

Daily Score

Water Intake + Break fast + Morning snack + Lunch + Afternoon snack + Dinner + Physical Activity = ( )

+13 to +16 Excellent
+9 to +12.9 Very Good
+5 to +8.9 Good
+1 to +4.9 Neutral
0 to -4.9 Poor
-5 to -8.9 Very Poor
-9 to -15 Critical

Hydration Scoring Scale

Water Intake (per day)*	Score
≥ 2.0 to 2.5 liters	2
1.5 to 2 liters	1
1 to 1.5 liters	0
0 to 1 liters	-1

Food Scoring Scale

Meal Quality	Score
Meal does not exist	1
Healthy and in reasonable quantity	2
Healthy but in excess	1
Neutral meal	0
Unhealthy meal	-1
Unhealthy and in excess	-2
Includes ice cream, cakes, soft drinks, or French fries	-1 per item

Physical Activity Scoring Scale

Activity Type	Score
Walking – 15 minutes	1
Running – 10 minutes	1
Other intense activities – 10 minutes	1
Sitting – every 2 hours continuously	-1

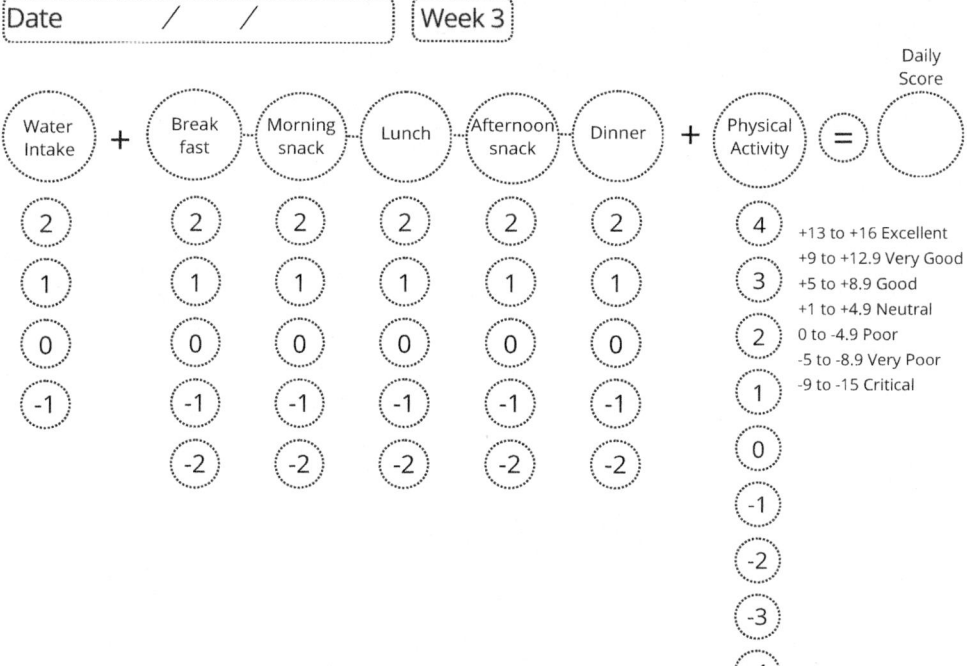

Daily Score

Water Intake + Break fast · Morning snack · Lunch · Afternoon snack · Dinner + Physical Activity = ( )

+13 to +16 Excellent
+9 to +12.9 Very Good
+5 to +8.9 Good
+1 to +4.9 Neutral
0 to -4.9 Poor
-5 to -8.9 Very Poor
-9 to -15 Critical

Hydration Scoring Scale

Water Intake (per day)*	Score
≥ 2.0 to 2.5 liters	2
1.5 to 2 liters	1
1 to 1.5 liters	0
0 to 1 liters	-1

Food Scoring Scale

Meal Quality	Score
Meal does not exist	1
Healthy and in reasonable quantity	2
Healthy but in excess	1
Neutral meal	0
Unhealthy meal	-1
Unhealthy and in excess	-2
Includes ice cream, cakes, soft drinks, or French fries	-1 per item

Physical Activity Scoring Scale

Activity Type	Score
Walking – 15 minutes	1
Running – 10 minutes	1
Other intense activities – 10 minutes	1
Sitting – every 2 hours continuously	-1

Date ____ / ____ / ____   Week 3

Daily
Score

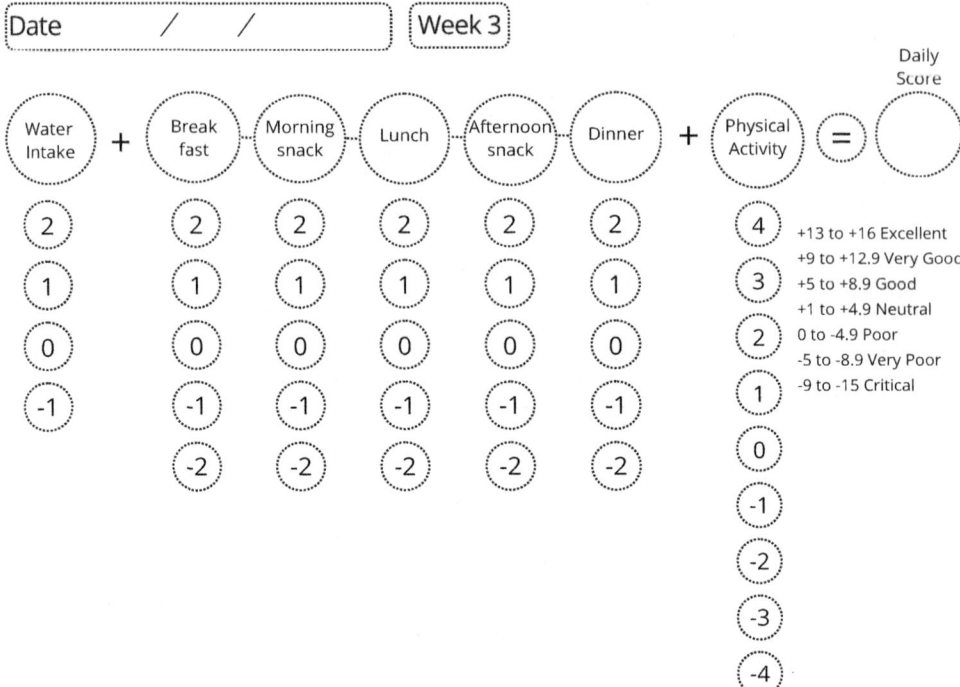

Water Intake	+	Break fast	Morning snack	Lunch	Afternoon snack	Dinner	+	Physical Activity	=	

+13 to +16 Excellent
+9 to +12.9 Very Good
+5 to +8.9 Good
+1 to +4.9 Neutral
0 to -4.9 Poor
-5 to -8.9 Very Poor
-9 to -15 Critical

End of Week 3 – Weekly Summary

Week 3 complete! What once felt like effort is now becoming habit. Keep going — real transformation is built one consistent day at a time.

Date ___ / ___ / ___   Week 4

Daily Score

(Water Intake) + (Break fast) (Morning snack) (Lunch) (Afternoon snack) (Dinner) + (Physical Activity) = ( )

Water Intake	Break fast	Morning snack	Lunch	Afternoon snack	Dinner	Physical Activity	
2	2	2	2	2	2	4	+13 to +16 Excellent
1	1	1	1	1	1	3	+9 to +12.9 Very Good
0	0	0	0	0	0	2	+5 to +8.9 Good
-1	-1	-1	-1	-1	-1	1	+1 to +4.9 Neutral
	-2	-2	-2	-2	-2	0	0 to -4.9 Poor
						-1	-5 to -8.9 Very Poor
						-2	-9 to -15 Critical
						-3	
						-4	

Hydration Scoring Scale

Water Intake (per day)*	Score
≥ 2.0 to 2.5 liters	2
1.5 to 2 liters	1
1 to 1.5 liters	0
0 to 1 liters	-1

Food Scoring Scale

Meal Quality	Score
Meal does not exist	1
Healthy and in reasonable quantity	2
Healthy but in excess	1
Neutral meal	0
Unhealthy meal	-1
Unhealthy and in excess	-2
Includes ice cream, cakes, soft drinks, or French fries	-1 per item

Physical Activity Scoring Scale

Activity Type	Score
Walking – 15 minutes	1
Running – 10 minutes	1
Other intense activities – 10 minutes	1
Sitting – every 2 hours continuously	-1

Date ____ / ____ / ____   Week 4

Water Intake + Break fast · Morning snack · Lunch · Afternoon snack · Dinner + Physical Activity = Daily Score

Water Intake: 2, 1, 0, -1

Break fast: 2, 1, 0, -1, -2

Morning snack: 2, 1, 0, -1, -2

Lunch: 2, 1, 0, -1, -2

Afternoon snack: 2, 1, 0, -1, -2

Dinner: 2, 1, 0, -1, -2

Physical Activity: 4, 3, 2, 1, 0, -1, -2, -3, -4

+13 to +16 Excellent
+9 to +12.9 Very Good
+5 to +8.9 Good
+1 to +4.9 Neutral
0 to -4.9 Poor
-5 to -8.9 Very Poor
-9 to -15 Critical

Hydration Scoring Scale

Water Intake (per day)*	Score
≥ 2.0 to 2.5 liters	2
1.5 to 2 liters	1
1 to 1.5 liters	0
0 to 1 liters	-1

Food Scoring Scale

Meal Quality	Score
Meal does not exist	1
Healthy and in reasonable quantity	2
Healthy but in excess	1
Neutral meal	0
Unhealthy meal	-1
Unhealthy and in excess	-2
Includes ice cream, cakes, soft drinks, or French fries	-1 per item

Physical Activity Scoring Scale

Activity Type	Score
Walking – 15 minutes	1
Running – 10 minutes	1
Other intense activities – 10 minutes	1
Sitting – every 2 hours continuously	-1

| Date / / | Week 4 |

Daily Score

(Water Intake) + (Break fast) (Morning snack) (Lunch) (Afternoon snack) (Dinner) + (Physical Activity) = ( )

Water Intake	Break fast	Morning snack	Lunch	Afternoon snack	Dinner	Physical Activity	
2	2	2	2	2	2	4	+13 to +16 Excellent
1	1	1	1	1	1	3	+9 to +12.9 Very Good
0	0	0	0	0	0	2	+5 to +8.9 Good
-1	-1	-1	-1	-1	-1	1	+1 to +4.9 Neutral
	-2	-2	-2	-2	-2	0	0 to -4.9 Poor
						-1	-5 to -8.9 Very Poor
						-2	-9 to -15 Critical
						-3	
						-4	

Hydration Scoring Scale

Water Intake (per day)*	Score
≥ 2.0 to 2.5 liters	2
1.5 to 2 liters	1
1 to 1.5 liters	0
0 to 1 liters	-1

Food Scoring Scale

Meal Quality	Score
Meal does not exist	1
Healthy and in reasonable quantity	2
Healthy but in excess	1
Neutral meal	0
Unhealthy meal	-1
Unhealthy and in excess	-2
Includes ice cream, cakes, soft drinks, or French fries	-1 per item

Physical Activity Scoring Scale

Activity Type	Score
Walking – 15 minutes	1
Running – 10 minutes	1
Other intense activities – 10 minutes	1
Sitting – every 2 hours continuously	-1

Date	/	/		Week 4

Daily Score

(Water Intake) + (Break fast) (Morning snack) (Lunch) (Afternoon snack) (Dinner) + (Physical Activity) = ( )

Water Intake	Break fast	Morning snack	Lunch	Afternoon snack	Dinner	Physical Activity	
2	2	2	2	2	2	4	+13 to +16 Excellent
1	1	1	1	1	1	3	+9 to +12.9 Very Good
0	0	0	0	0	0	2	+5 to +8.9 Good
-1	-1	-1	-1	-1	-1	1	+1 to +4.9 Neutral
	-2	-2	-2	-2	-2	0	0 to -4.9 Poor
						-1	-5 to -8.9 Very Poor
						-2	-9 to -15 Critical
						-3	
						-4	

Hydration Scoring Scale

Water Intake (per day)*	Score
≥ 2.0 to 2.5 liters	2
1.5 to 2 liters	1
1 to 1.5 liters	0
0 to 1 liters	-1

Food Scoring Scale

Meal Quality	Score
Meal does not exist	1
Healthy and in reasonable quantity	2
Healthy but in excess	1
Neutral meal	0
Unhealthy meal	-1
Unhealthy and in excess	-2
Includes ice cream, cakes, soft drinks, or French fries	-1 per item

Physical Activity Scoring Scale

Activity Type	Score
Walking – 15 minutes	1
Running – 10 minutes	1
Other intense activities – 10 minutes	1
Sitting – every 2 hours continuously	-1

Date   /   /   Week 4

Daily Score

(Water Intake) + (Break fast) (Morning snack) (Lunch) (Afternoon snack) (Dinner) + (Physical Activity) = ( )

Water Intake: 2, 1, 0, -1

Break fast: 2, 1, 0, -1, -2

Morning snack: 2, 1, 0, -1, -2

Lunch: 2, 1, 0, -1, -2

Afternoon snack: 2, 1, 0, -1, -2

Dinner: 2, 1, 0, -1, -2

Physical Activity: 4, 3, 2, 1, 0, -1, -2, -3, -4

+13 to +16 Excellent
+9 to +12.9 Very Good
+5 to +8.9 Good
+1 to +4.9 Neutral
0 to -4.9 Poor
-5 to -8.9 Very Poor
-9 to -15 Critical

Hydration Scoring Scale

Water Intake (per day)*	Score
≥ 2.0 to 2.5 liters	2
1.5 to 2 liters	1
1 to 1.5 liters	0
0 to 1 liters	-1

Food Scoring Scale

Meal Quality	Score
Meal does not exist	1
Healthy and in reasonable quantity	2
Healthy but in excess	1
Neutral meal	0
Unhealthy meal	-1
Unhealthy and in excess	-2
Includes ice cream, cakes, soft drinks, or French fries	-1 per item

Physical Activity Scoring Scale

Activity Type	Score
Walking – 15 minutes	1
Running – 10 minutes	1
Other intense activities – 10 minutes	1
Sitting – every 2 hours continuously	-1

53

Date	/	/		Week 4

(Water Intake) + (Break fast) (Morning snack) (Lunch) (Afternoon snack) (Dinner) + (Physical Activity) = (Daily Score)

Water Intake	Break fast	Morning snack	Lunch	Afternoon snack	Dinner	Physical Activity
2	2	2	2	2	2	4
1	1	1	1	1	1	3
0	0	0	0	0	0	2
-1	-1	-1	-1	-1	-1	1
	-2	-2	-2	-2	-2	0
						-1
						-2
						-3
						-4

+13 to +16 Excellent
+9 to +12.9 Very Good
+5 to +8.9 Good
+1 to +4.9 Neutral
0 to -4.9 Poor
-5 to -8.9 Very Poor
-9 to -15 Critical

Hydration Scoring Scale

Water Intake (per day)*	Score
≥ 2.0 to 2.5 liters	2
1.5 to 2 liters	1
1 to 1.5 liters	0
0 to 1 liters	-1

Food Scoring Scale

Meal Quality	Score
Meal does not exist	1
Healthy and in reasonable quantity	2
Healthy but in excess	1
Neutral meal	0
Unhealthy meal	-1
Unhealthy and in excess	-2
Includes ice cream, cakes, soft drinks, or French fries	-1 per item

Physical Activity Scoring Scale

Activity Type	Score
Walking – 15 minutes	1
Running – 10 minutes	1
Other intense activities – 10 minutes	1
Sitting – every 2 hours continuously	-1

Date / /	Week 4

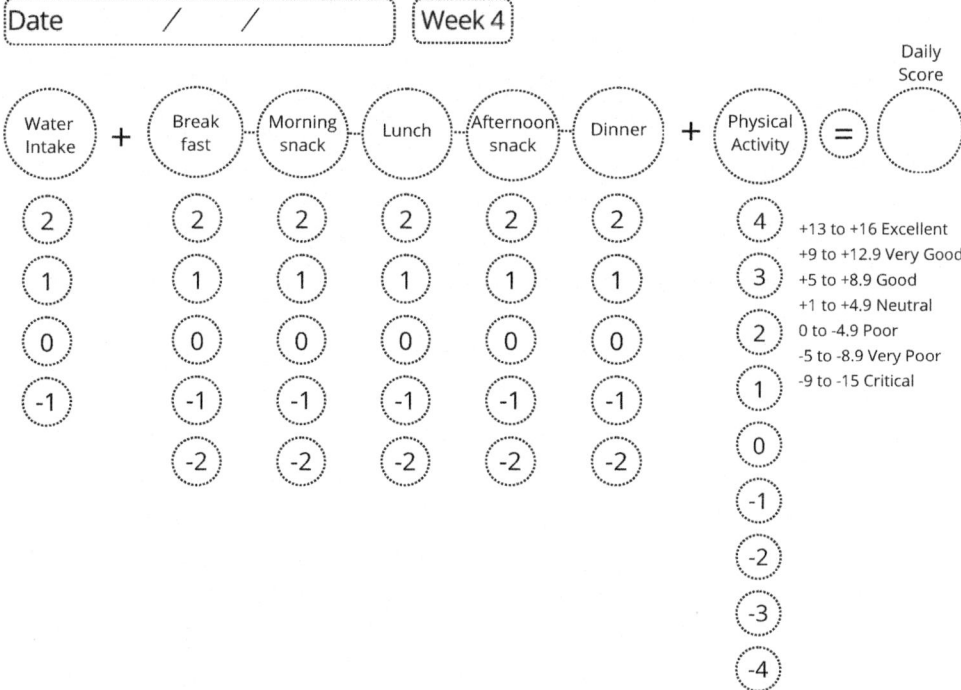

Daily Score

Water Intake + Break fast — Morning snack — Lunch — Afternoon snack — Dinner + Physical Activity = ( )

+13 to +16 Excellent
+9 to +12.9 Very Good
+5 to +8.9 Good
+1 to +4.9 Neutral
0 to -4.9 Poor
-5 to -8.9 Very Poor
-9 to -15 Critical

End of Week 4 – Weekly Summary

One month down! You've proven to yourself that you can commit and stay focused. Keep the momentum — you're not just changing your body, you're building a new lifestyle.

Daily Score

(Water Intake) + (Break fast) (Morning snack) (Lunch) (Afternoon snack) (Dinner) + (Physical Activity) = ( )

Water Intake	Breakfast	Morning snack	Lunch	Afternoon snack	Dinner	Physical Activity
2	2	2	2	2	2	4
1	1	1	1	1	1	3
0	0	0	0	0	0	2
-1	-1	-1	-1	-1	-1	1
	-2	-2	-2	-2	-2	0
						-1
						-2
						-3
						-4

+13 to +16 Excellent
+9 to +12.9 Very Good
+5 to +8.9 Good
+1 to +4.9 Neutral
0 to -4.9 Poor
-5 to -8.9 Very Poor
-9 to -15 Critical

Hydration Scoring Scale

Water Intake (per day)*	Score
≥ 2.0 to 2.5 liters	2
1.5 to 2 liters	1
1 to 1.5 liters	0
0 to 1 liters	-1

Food Scoring Scale

Meal Quality	Score
Meal does not exist	1
Healthy and in reasonable quantity	2
Healthy but in excess	1
Neutral meal	0
Unhealthy meal	-1
Unhealthy and in excess	-2
Includes ice cream, cakes, soft drinks, or French fries	-1 per item

Physical Activity Scoring Scale

Activity Type	Score
Walking – 15 minutes	1
Running – 10 minutes	1
Other intense activities – 10 minutes	1
Sitting – every 2 hours continuously	-1

Daily Score

(Water Intake) + (Break fast) (Morning snack) (Lunch) (Afternoon snack) (Dinner) + (Physical Activity) = ( )

Water Intake	Break fast	Morning snack	Lunch	Afternoon snack	Dinner		Physical Activity	
2	2	2	2	2	2		4	+13 to +16 Excellent
1	1	1	1	1	1		3	+9 to +12.9 Very Good
0	0	0	0	0	0		2	+5 to +8.9 Good
-1	-1	-1	-1	-1	-1		1	+1 to +4.9 Neutral
	-2	-2	-2	-2	-2		0	0 to -4.9 Poor
							-1	-5 to -8.9 Very Poor
							-2	-9 to -15 Critical
							-3	
							-4	

Hydration Scoring Scale

Water Intake (per day)*	Score
≥ 2.0 to 2.5 liters	2
1.5 to 2 liters	1
1 to 1.5 liters	0
0 to 1 liters	-1

Food Scoring Scale

Meal Quality	Score
Meal does not exist	1
Healthy and in reasonable quantity	2
Healthy but in excess	1
Neutral meal	0
Unhealthy meal	-1
Unhealthy and in excess	-2
Includes ice cream, cakes, soft drinks, or French fries	-1 per item

Physical Activity Scoring Scale

Activity Type	Score
Walking – 15 minutes	1
Running – 10 minutes	1
Other intense activities – 10 minutes	1
Sitting – every 2 hours continuously	-1

Water Intake + Break fast · Morning snack · Lunch · Afternoon snack · Dinner + Physical Activity = Daily Score

Water Intake	Breakfast	Morning snack	Lunch	Afternoon snack	Dinner	Physical Activity
2	2	2	2	2	2	4
1	1	1	1	1	1	3
0	0	0	0	0	0	2
-1	-1	-1	-1	-1	-1	1
	-2	-2	-2	-2	-2	0
						-1
						-2
						-3
						-4

+13 to +16 Excellent
+9 to +12.9 Very Good
+5 to +8.9 Good
+1 to +4.9 Neutral
0 to -4.9 Poor
-5 to -8.9 Very Poor
-9 to -15 Critical

Hydration Scoring Scale

Water Intake (per day)*	Score
≥ 2.0 to 2.5 liters	2
1.5 to 2 liters	1
1 to 1.5 liters	0
0 to 1 liters	-1

Food Scoring Scale

Meal Quality	Score
Meal does not exist	1
Healthy and in reasonable quantity	2
Healthy but in excess	1
Neutral meal	0
Unhealthy meal	-1
Unhealthy and in excess	-2
Includes ice cream, cakes, soft drinks, or French fries	-1 per item

Physical Activity Scoring Scale

Activity Type	Score
Walking – 15 minutes	1
Running – 10 minutes	1
Other intense activities – 10 minutes	1
Sitting – every 2 hours continuously	-1

Daily Score

Water Intake + Break fast   Morning snack   Lunch   Afternoon snack   Dinner + Physical Activity = ○

Water Intake	Breakfast	Morning snack	Lunch	Afternoon snack	Dinner	Physical Activity
2	2	2	2	2	2	4
1	1	1	1	1	1	3
0	0	0	0	0	0	2
-1	-1	-1	-1	-1	-1	1
	-2	-2	-2	-2	-2	0
						-1
						-2
						-3
						-4

+13 to +16 Excellent
+9 to +12.9 Very Good
+5 to +8.9 Good
+1 to +4.9 Neutral
0 to -4.9 Poor
-5 to -8.9 Very Poor
-9 to -15 Critical

Hydration Scoring Scale

Water Intake (per day)*	Score
≥ 2.0 to 2.5 liters	2
1.5 to 2 liters	1
1 to 1.5 liters	0
0 to 1 liters	-1

Food Scoring Scale

Meal Quality	Score
Meal does not exist	1
Healthy and in reasonable quantity	2
Healthy but in excess	1
Neutral meal	0
Unhealthy meal	-1
Unhealthy and in excess	-2
Includes ice cream, cakes, soft drinks, or French fries	-1 per item

Physical Activity Scoring Scale

Activity Type	Score
Walking – 15 minutes	1
Running – 10 minutes	1
Other intense activities – 10 minutes	1
Sitting – every 2 hours continuously	-1

Daily Score

(Water Intake) + (Break fast) (Morning snack) (Lunch) (Afternoon snack) (Dinner) + (Physical Activity) = ( )

Water Intake	Break fast	Morning snack	Lunch	Afternoon snack	Dinner	Physical Activity
2	2	2	2	2	2	4
1	1	1	1	1	1	3
0	0	0	0	0	0	2
-1	-1	-1	-1	-1	-1	1
	-2	-2	-2	-2	-2	0
						-1
						-2
						-3
						-4

+13 to +16 Excellent
+9 to +12.9 Very Good
+5 to +8.9 Good
+1 to +4.9 Neutral
0 to -4.9 Poor
-5 to -8.9 Very Poor
-9 to -15 Critical

Hydration Scoring Scale

Water Intake (per day)*	Score
≥ 2.0 to 2.5 liters	2
1.5 to 2 liters	1
1 to 1.5 liters	0
0 to 1 liters	-1

Food Scoring Scale

Meal Quality	Score
Meal does not exist	1
Healthy and in reasonable quantity	2
Healthy but in excess	1
Neutral meal	0
Unhealthy meal	-1
Unhealthy and in excess	-2
Includes ice cream, cakes, soft drinks, or French fries	-1 per item

Physical Activity Scoring Scale

Activity Type	Score
Walking – 15 minutes	1
Running – 10 minutes	1
Other intense activities – 10 minutes	1
Sitting – every 2 hours continuously	-1

Date	/	/		Week 5

Water Intake	+	Break fast	Morning snack	Lunch	Afternoon snack	Dinner	+	Physical Activity	=	Daily Score

Water Intake	Break fast	Morning snack	Lunch	Afternoon snack	Dinner	Physical Activity	
2	2	2	2	2	2	4	+13 to +16 Excellent
1	1	1	1	1	1	3	+9 to +12.9 Very Good
0	0	0	0	0	0	2	+5 to +8.9 Good
-1	-1	-1	-1	-1	-1	1	+1 to +4.9 Neutral
	-2	-2	-2	-2	-2	0	0 to -4.9 Poor
						-1	-5 to -8.9 Very Poor
						-2	-9 to -15 Critical
						-3	
						-4	

Hydration Scoring Scale

Water Intake (per day)*	Score
≥ 2.0 to 2.5 liters	2
1.5 to 2 liters	1
1 to 1.5 liters	0
0 to 1 liters	-1

Food Scoring Scale

Meal Quality	Score
Meal does not exist	1
Healthy and in reasonable quantity	2
Healthy but in excess	1
Neutral meal	0
Unhealthy meal	-1
Unhealthy and in excess	-2
Includes ice cream, cakes, soft drinks, or French fries	-1 per item

Physical Activity Scoring Scale

Activity Type	Score
Walking – 15 minutes	1
Running – 10 minutes	1
Other intense activities – 10 minutes	1
Sitting – every 2 hours continuously	-1

Date	/	/		Week 5

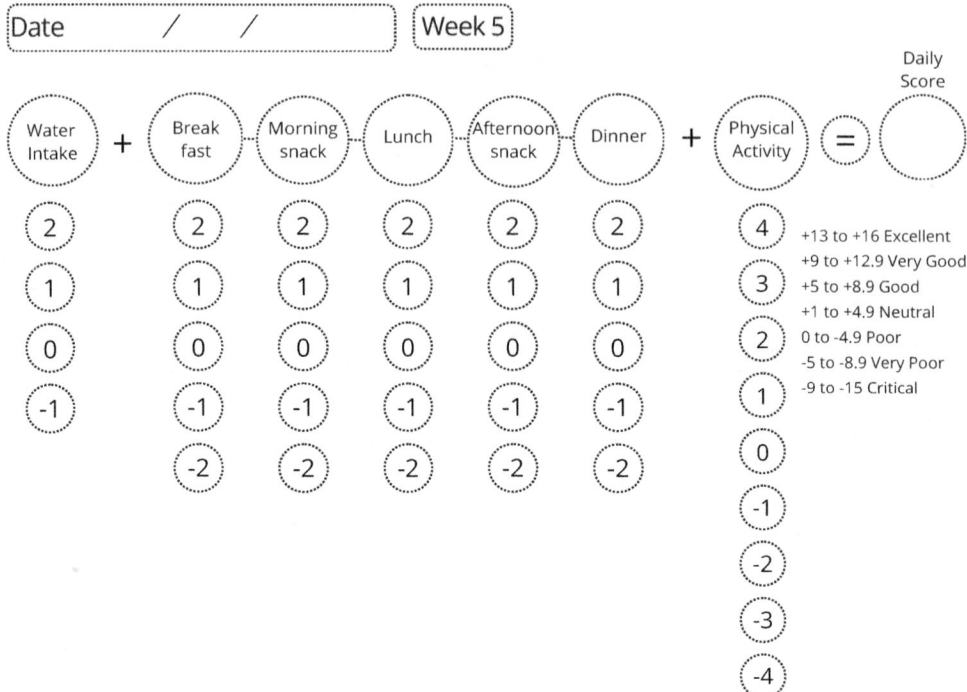

Daily Score

| Water Intake | + | Break fast | Morning snack | Lunch | Afternoon snack | Dinner | + | Physical Activity | = | |

2	2	2	2	2	2	4	+13 to +16 Excellent
1	1	1	1	1	1	3	+9 to +12.9 Very Good
0	0	0	0	0	0	2	+5 to +8.9 Good
-1	-1	-1	-1	-1	-1	1	+1 to +4.9 Neutral
	-2	-2	-2	-2	-2	0	0 to -4.9 Poor
						-1	-5 to -8.9 Very Poor
						-2	-9 to -15 Critical
						-3	
						-4	

End of Week 5 – Weekly Summary

Five weeks in — you're not just forming habits, you're building a lifestyle. Keep showing up for yourself.

Daily Score

Water Intake $+$ Break fast   Morning snack   Lunch   Afternoon snack   Dinner $+$ Physical Activity $=$ ◯

Water Intake	Break fast	Morning snack	Lunch	Afternoon snack	Dinner	Physical Activity	
2	2	2	2	2	2	4	+13 to +16 Excellent
1	1	1	1	1	1	3	+9 to +12.9 Very Good
0	0	0	0	0	0	2	+5 to +8.9 Good
-1	-1	-1	-1	-1	-1	1	+1 to +4.9 Neutral
	-2	-2	-2	-2	-2	0	0 to -4.9 Poor
						-1	-5 to -8.9 Very Poor
						-2	-9 to -15 Critical
						-3	
						-4	

Hydration Scoring Scale

Water Intake (per day)*	Score
≥ 2.0 to 2.5 liters	2
1.5 to 2 liters	1
1 to 1.5 liters	0
0 to 1 liters	-1

Food Scoring Scale

Meal Quality	Score
Meal does not exist	1
Healthy and in reasonable quantity	2
Healthy but in excess	1
Neutral meal	0
Unhealthy meal	-1
Unhealthy and in excess	-2
Includes ice cream, cakes, soft drinks, or French fries	-1 per item

Physical Activity Scoring Scale

Activity Type	Score
Walking – 15 minutes	1
Running – 10 minutes	1
Other intense activities – 10 minutes	1
Sitting – every 2 hours continuously	-1

Daily Score

| Water Intake | + | Break fast | Morning snack | Lunch | Afternoon snack | Dinner | + | Physical Activity | = | |

Water Intake column: 2, 1, 0, -1

Breakfast: 2, 1, 0, -1, -2

Morning snack: 2, 1, 0, -1, -2

Lunch: 2, 1, 0, -1, -2

Afternoon snack: 2, 1, 0, -1, -2

Dinner: 2, 1, 0, -1, -2

Physical Activity: 4, 3, 2, 1, 0, -1, -2, -3, -4

+13 to +16 Excellent
+9 to +12.9 Very Good
+5 to +8.9 Good
+1 to +4.9 Neutral
0 to -4.9 Poor
-5 to -8.9 Very Poor
-9 to -15 Critical

Hydration Scoring Scale

Water Intake (per day)*	Score
≥ 2.0 to 2.5 liters	2
1.5 to 2 liters	1
1 to 1.5 liters	0
0 to 1 liters	-1

Food Scoring Scale

Meal Quality	Score
Meal does not exist	1
Healthy and in reasonable quantity	2
Healthy but in excess	1
Neutral meal	0
Unhealthy meal	-1
Unhealthy and in excess	-2
Includes ice cream, cakes, soft drinks, or French fries	-1 per item

Physical Activity Scoring Scale

Activity Type	Score
Walking – 15 minutes	1
Running – 10 minutes	1
Other intense activities – 10 minutes	1
Sitting – every 2 hours continuously	-1

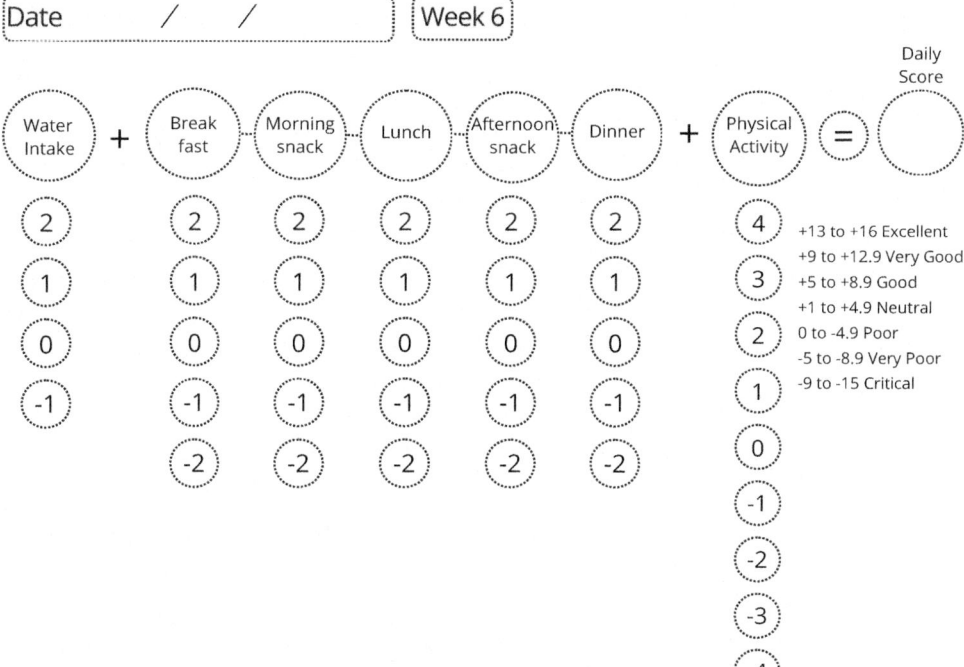

Date _____ / _____ / _____   Week 6

Daily Score

Water Intake + Break fast · Morning snack · Lunch · Afternoon snack · Dinner + Physical Activity = ( )

Water Intake: 2, 1, 0, -1

Break fast: 2, 1, 0, -1, -2

Morning snack: 2, 1, 0, -1, -2

Lunch: 2, 1, 0, -1, -2

Afternoon snack: 2, 1, 0, -1, -2

Dinner: 2, 1, 0, -1, -2

Physical Activity: 4, 3, 2, 1, 0, -1, -2, -3, -4

+13 to +16 Excellent
+9 to +12.9 Very Good
+5 to +8.9 Good
+1 to +4.9 Neutral
0 to -4.9 Poor
-5 to -8.9 Very Poor
-9 to -15 Critical

Hydration Scoring Scale

Water Intake (per day)*	Score
≥ 2.0 to 2.5 liters	2
1.5 to 2 liters	1
1 to 1.5 liters	0
0 to 1 liters	-1

Food Scoring Scale

Meal Quality	Score
Meal does not exist	1
Healthy and in reasonable quantity	2
Healthy but in excess	1
Neutral meal	0
Unhealthy meal	-1
Unhealthy and in excess	-2
Includes ice cream, cakes, soft drinks, or French fries	-1 per item

Physical Activity Scoring Scale

Activity Type	Score
Walking – 15 minutes	1
Running – 10 minutes	1
Other intense activities – 10 minutes	1
Sitting – every 2 hours continuously	-1

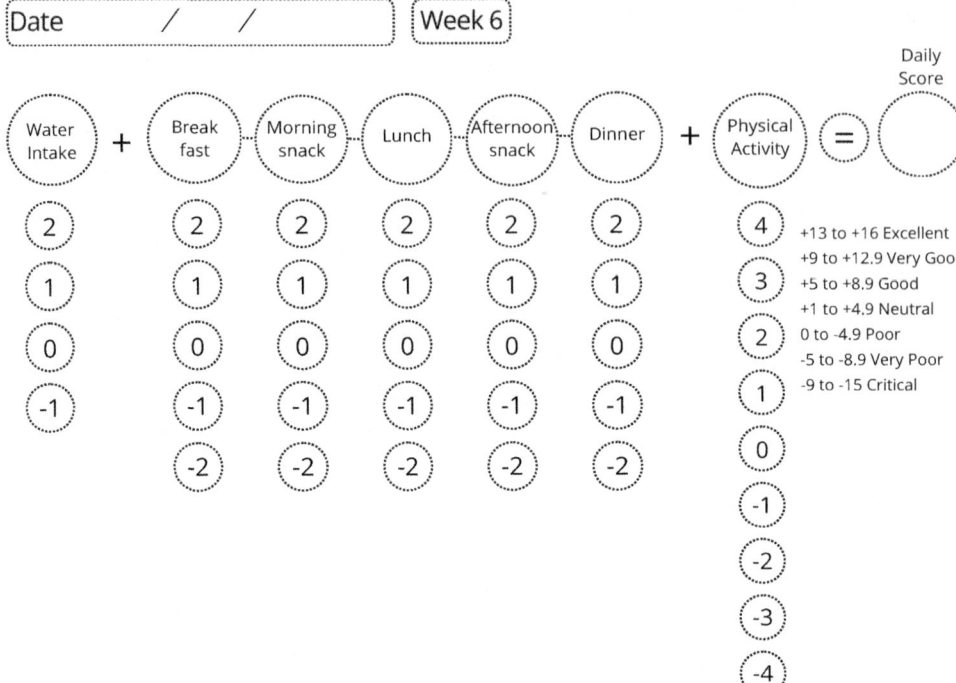

Hydration Scoring Scale	
Water Intake (per day)*	**Score**
≥ 2.0 to 2.5 liters	2
1.5 to 2 liters	1
1 to 1.5 liters	0
0 to 1 liters	-1

Food Scoring Scale	
Meal Quality	**Score**
Meal does not exist	1
Healthy and in reasonable quantity	2
Healthy but in excess	1
Neutral meal	0
Unhealthy meal	-1
Unhealthy and in excess	-2
Includes ice cream, cakes, soft drinks, or French fries	-1 per item

Physical Activity Scoring Scale	
Activity Type	**Score**
Walking – 15 minutes	1
Running – 10 minutes	1
Other intense activities – 10 minutes	1
Sitting – every 2 hours continuously	-1

Daily Score

(Water Intake) + (Break fast) (Morning snack) (Lunch) (Afternoon snack) (Dinner) + (Physical Activity) = ( )

Water Intake	Break fast	Morning snack	Lunch	Afternoon snack	Dinner	Physical Activity
2	2	2	2	2	2	4
1	1	1	1	1	1	3
0	0	0	0	0	0	2
-1	-1	-1	-1	-1	-1	1
	-2	-2	-2	-2	-2	0
						-1
						-2
						-3
						-4

+13 to +16 Excellent
+9 to +12.9 Very Good
+5 to +8.9 Good
+1 to +4.9 Neutral
0 to -4.9 Poor
-5 to -8.9 Very Poor
-9 to -15 Critical

Hydration Scoring Scale

Water Intake (per day)*	Score
≥ 2.0 to 2.5 liters	2
1.5 to 2 liters	1
1 to 1.5 liters	0
0 to 1 liters	-1

Food Scoring Scale

Meal Quality	Score
Meal does not exist	1
Healthy and in reasonable quantity	2
Healthy but in excess	1
Neutral meal	0
Unhealthy meal	-1
Unhealthy and in excess	-2
Includes ice cream, cakes, soft drinks, or French fries	-1 per item

Physical Activity Scoring Scale

Activity Type	Score
Walking – 15 minutes	1
Running – 10 minutes	1
Other intense activities – 10 minutes	1
Sitting – every 2 hours continuously	-1

Daily Score

Water Intake + Break fast | Morning snack | Lunch | Afternoon snack | Dinner + Physical Activity = ( )

Water Intake: 2, 1, 0, -1

Breakfast: 2, 1, 0, -1, -2

Morning snack: 2, 1, 0, -1, -2

Lunch: 2, 1, 0, -1, -2

Afternoon snack: 2, 1, 0, -1, -2

Dinner: 2, 1, 0, -1, -2

Physical Activity: 4, 3, 2, 1, 0, -1, -2, -3, -4

+13 to +16 Excellent
+9 to +12.9 Very Good
+5 to +8.9 Good
+1 to +4.9 Neutral
0 to -4.9 Poor
-5 to -8.9 Very Poor
-9 to -15 Critical

Hydration Scoring Scale

Water Intake (per day)*	Score
≥ 2.0 to 2.5 liters	2
1.5 to 2 liters	1
1 to 1.5 liters	0
0 to 1 liters	-1

Food Scoring Scale

Meal Quality	Score
Meal does not exist	1
Healthy and in reasonable quantity	2
Healthy but in excess	1
Neutral meal	0
Unhealthy meal	-1
Unhealthy and in excess	-2
Includes ice cream, cakes, soft drinks, or French fries	-1 per item

Physical Activity Scoring Scale

Activity Type	Score
Walking – 15 minutes	1
Running – 10 minutes	1
Other intense activities – 10 minutes	1
Sitting – every 2 hours continuously	-1

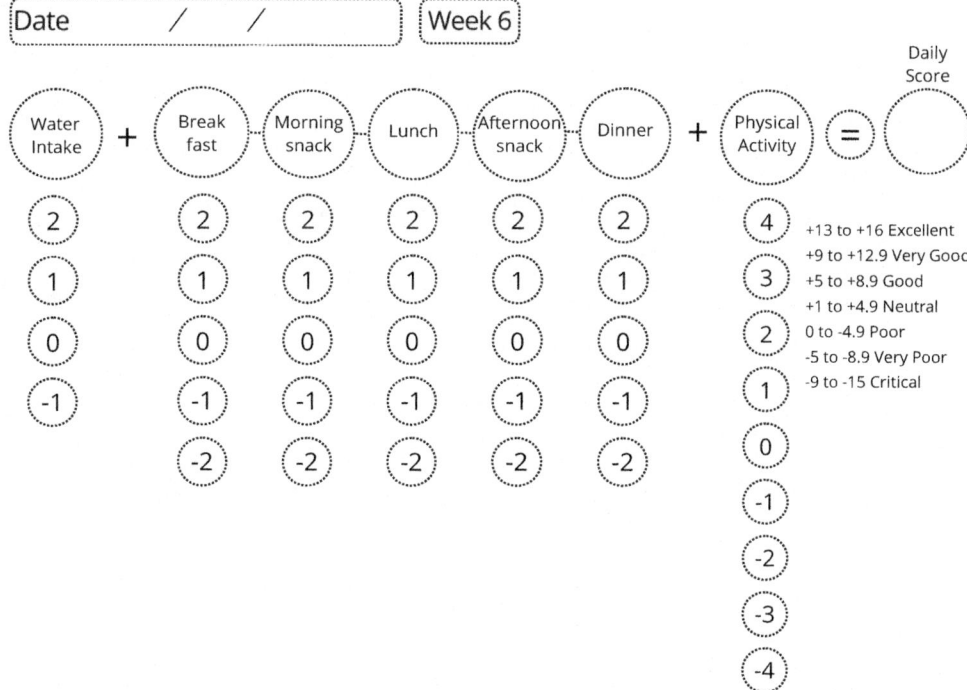

Date / /	Week 6

End of Week 6 – Weekly Summary

Six weeks of effort, discipline, and growth — the results are building, even if they're not all visible yet. Trust the process.

Water Intake	+	Break fast	Morning snack	Lunch	Afternoon snack	Dinner	+	Physical Activity	=	Daily Score
2		2	2	2	2	2		4		
1		1	1	1	1	1		3		
0		0	0	0	0	0		2		
-1		-1	-1	-1	-1	-1		1		
		-2	-2	-2	-2	-2		0		
								-1		
								-2		
								-3		
								-4		

+13 to +16 Excellent
+9 to +12.9 Very Good
+5 to +8.9 Good
+1 to +4.9 Neutral
0 to -4.9 Poor
-5 to -8.9 Very Poor
-9 to -15 Critical

Hydration Scoring Scale

Water Intake (per day)*	Score
≥ 2.0 to 2.5 liters	2
1.5 to 2 liters	1
1 to 1.5 liters	0
0 to 1 liters	-1

Food Scoring Scale

Meal Quality	Score
Meal does not exist	1
Healthy and in reasonable quantity	2
Healthy but in excess	1
Neutral meal	0
Unhealthy meal	-1
Unhealthy and in excess	-2
Includes ice cream, cakes, soft drinks, or French fries	-1 per item

Physical Activity Scoring Scale

Activity Type	Score
Walking – 15 minutes	1
Running – 10 minutes	1
Other intense activities – 10 minutes	1
Sitting – every 2 hours continuously	-1

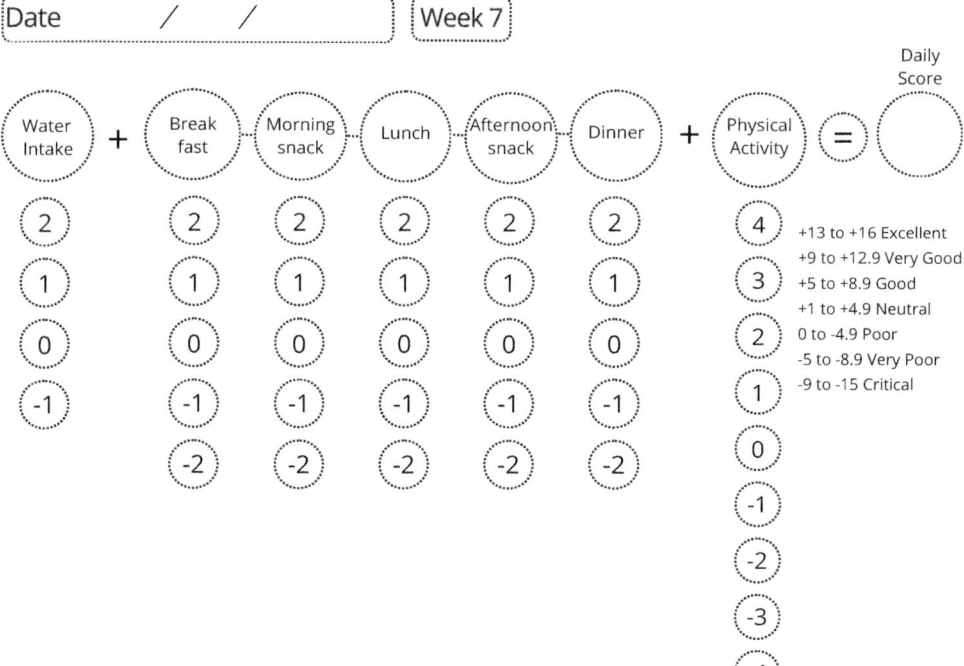

Daily Score

| Water Intake | + | Break fast | Morning snack | Lunch | Afternoon snack | Dinner | + | Physical Activity | = | |

+13 to +16 Excellent
+9 to +12.9 Very Good
+5 to +8.9 Good
+1 to +4.9 Neutral
0 to -4.9 Poor
-5 to -8.9 Very Poor
-9 to -15 Critical

Hydration Scoring Scale

Water Intake (per day)*	Score
≥ 2.0 to 2.5 liters	2
1.5 to 2 liters	1
1 to 1.5 liters	0
0 to 1 liters	-1

Food Scoring Scale

Meal Quality	Score
Meal does not exist	1
Healthy and in reasonable quantity	2
Healthy but in excess	1
Neutral meal	0
Unhealthy meal	-1
Unhealthy and in excess	-2
Includes ice cream, cakes, soft drinks, or French fries	-1 per item

Physical Activity Scoring Scale

Activity Type	Score
Walking – 15 minutes	1
Running – 10 minutes	1
Other intense activities – 10 minutes	1
Sitting – every 2 hours continuously	-1

Daily Score

(Water Intake) + (Break fast) (Morning snack) (Lunch) (Afternoon snack) (Dinner) + (Physical Activity) = ( )

Water Intake	Break fast	Morning snack	Lunch	Afternoon snack	Dinner	Physical Activity	
2	2	2	2	2	2	4	+13 to +16 Excellent
1	1	1	1	1	1	3	+9 to +12.9 Very Good
0	0	0	0	0	0	2	+5 to +8.9 Good
-1	-1	-1	-1	-1	-1	1	+1 to +4.9 Neutral
	-2	-2	-2	-2	-2	0	0 to -4.9 Poor
						-1	-5 to -8.9 Very Poor
						-2	-9 to -15 Critical
						-3	
						-4	

Hydration Scoring Scale

Water Intake (per day)*	Score
≥ 2.0 to 2.5 liters	2
1.5 to 2 liters	1
1 to 1.5 liters	0
0 to 1 liters	-1

Food Scoring Scale

Meal Quality	Score
Meal does not exist	1
Healthy and in reasonable quantity	2
Healthy but in excess	1
Neutral meal	0
Unhealthy meal	-1
Unhealthy and in excess	-2
Includes ice cream, cakes, soft drinks, or French fries	-1 per item

Physical Activity Scoring Scale

Activity Type	Score
Walking – 15 minutes	1
Running – 10 minutes	1
Other intense activities – 10 minutes	1
Sitting – every 2 hours continuously	-1

| Date | / / | Week 7 |

Daily Score

| Water Intake | + | Break fast | Morning snack | Lunch | Afternoon snack | Dinner | + | Physical Activity | = | ( ) |

Water Intake	Break fast	Morning snack	Lunch	Afternoon snack	Dinner	Physical Activity
2	2	2	2	2	2	4
1	1	1	1	1	1	3
0	0	0	0	0	0	2
-1	-1	-1	-1	-1	-1	1
	-2	-2	-2	-2	-2	0
						-1
						-2
						-3
						-4

+13 to +16 Excellent
+9 to +12.9 Very Good
+5 to +8.9 Good
+1 to +4.9 Neutral
0 to -4.9 Poor
-5 to -8.9 Very Poor
-9 to -15 Critical

Hydration Scoring Scale

Water Intake (per day)*	Score
≥ 2.0 to 2.5 liters	2
1.5 to 2 liters	1
1 to 1.5 liters	0
0 to 1 liters	-1

Food Scoring Scale

Meal Quality	Score
Meal does not exist	1
Healthy and in reasonable quantity	2
Healthy but in excess	1
Neutral meal	0
Unhealthy meal	-1
Unhealthy and in excess	-2
Includes ice cream, cakes, soft drinks, or French fries	-1 per item

Physical Activity Scoring Scale

Activity Type	Score
Walking – 15 minutes	1
Running – 10 minutes	1
Other intense activities – 10 minutes	1
Sitting – every 2 hours continuously	-1

Daily Score

(Water Intake) + (Break fast) (Morning snack) (Lunch) (Afternoon snack) (Dinner) + (Physical Activity) = ( )

Water Intake	Break fast	Morning snack	Lunch	Afternoon snack	Dinner	Physical Activity	
2	2	2	2	2	2	4	+13 to +16 Excellent
1	1	1	1	1	1	3	+9 to +12.9 Very Good
0	0	0	0	0	0	2	+5 to +8.9 Good
-1	-1	-1	-1	-1	-1	1	+1 to +4.9 Neutral
	-2	-2	-2	-2	-2	0	0 to -4.9 Poor
						-1	-5 to -8.9 Very Poor
						-2	-9 to -15 Critical
						-3	
						-4	

Hydration Scoring Scale

Water Intake (per day)*	Score
≥ 2.0 to 2.5 liters	2
1.5 to 2 liters	1
1 to 1.5 liters	0
0 to 1 liters	-1

Food Scoring Scale

Meal Quality	Score
Meal does not exist	1
Healthy and in reasonable quantity	2
Healthy but in excess	1
Neutral meal	0
Unhealthy meal	-1
Unhealthy and in excess	-2
Includes ice cream, cakes, soft drinks, or French fries	-1 per item

Physical Activity Scoring Scale

Activity Type	Score
Walking – 15 minutes	1
Running – 10 minutes	1
Other intense activities – 10 minutes	1
Sitting – every 2 hours continuously	-1

Date ____ / ____ / ____   Week 7

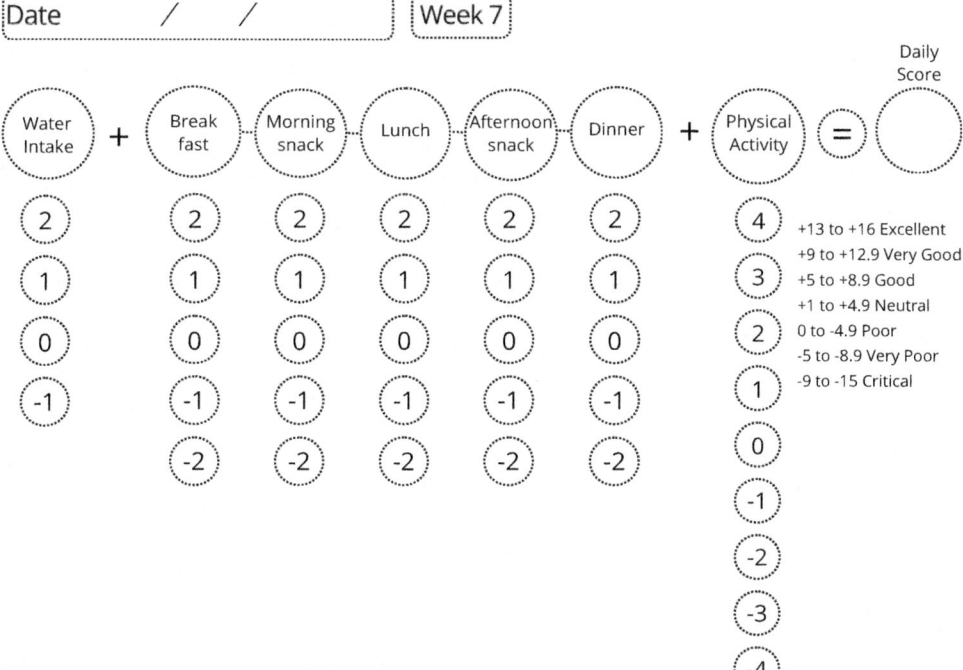

Daily Score

Water Intake + Break fast · Morning snack · Lunch · Afternoon snack · Dinner + Physical Activity = ◯

Water Intake	Break fast	Morning snack	Lunch	Afternoon snack	Dinner	Physical Activity	
2	2	2	2	2	2	4	+13 to +16 Excellent
1	1	1	1	1	1	3	+9 to +12.9 Very Good
0	0	0	0	0	0	2	+5 to +8.9 Good
-1	-1	-1	-1	-1	-1	1	+1 to +4.9 Neutral
	-2	-2	-2	-2	-2	0	0 to -4.9 Poor
						-1	-5 to -8.9 Very Poor
						-2	-9 to -15 Critical
						-3	
						-4	

Hydration Scoring Scale

Water Intake (per day)*	Score
≥ 2.0 to 2.5 liters	2
1.5 to 2 liters	1
1 to 1.5 liters	0
0 to 1 liters	-1

Food Scoring Scale

Meal Quality	Score
Meal does not exist	1
Healthy and in reasonable quantity	2
Healthy but in excess	1
Neutral meal	0
Unhealthy meal	-1
Unhealthy and in excess	-2
Includes ice cream, cakes, soft drinks, or French fries	-1 per item

Physical Activity Scoring Scale

Activity Type	Score
Walking – 15 minutes	1
Running – 10 minutes	1
Other intense activities – 10 minutes	1
Sitting – every 2 hours continuously	-1

Date	/	/		Week 7

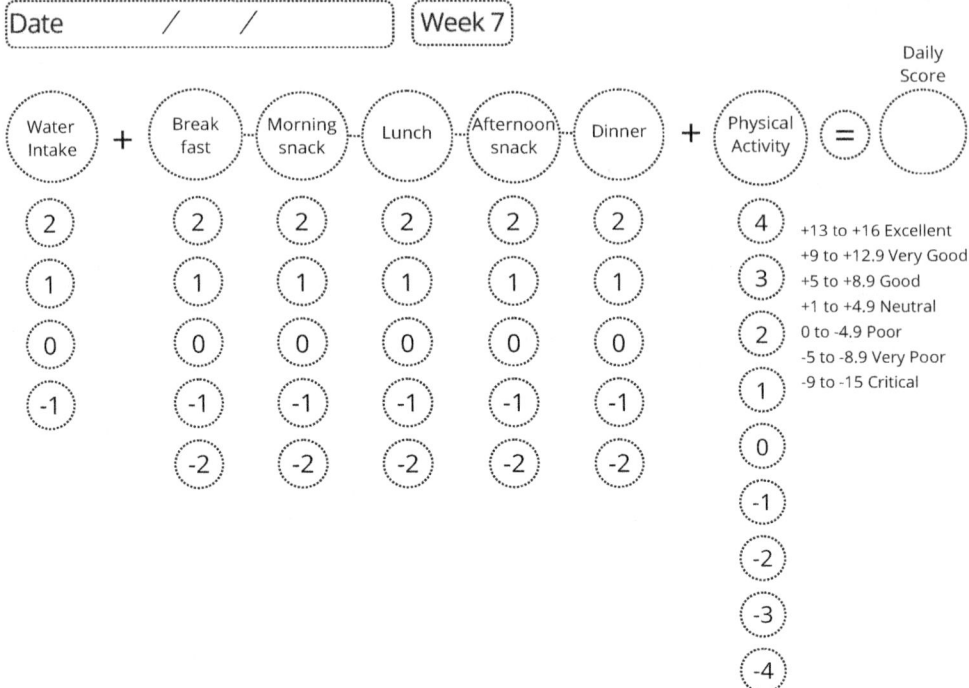

End of Week 7 – Weekly Summary

Week 7 complete — you're not just changing habits, you're changing who you are. Keep moving forward.

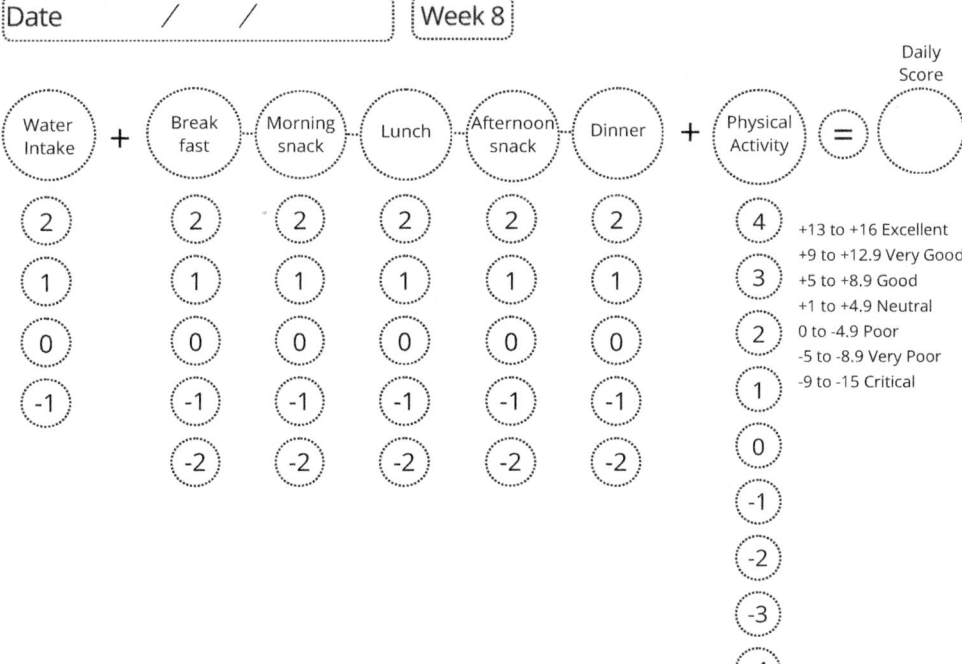

Date ___ / ___ / ___   Week 8

Daily Score

Water Intake + Break fast | Morning snack | Lunch | Afternoon snack | Dinner + Physical Activity = ( )

Water Intake: 2, 1, 0, -1

Breakfast: 2, 1, 0, -1, -2
Morning snack: 2, 1, 0, -1, -2
Lunch: 2, 1, 0, -1, -2
Afternoon snack: 2, 1, 0, -1, -2
Dinner: 2, 1, 0, -1, -2

Physical Activity: 4, 3, 2, 1, 0, -1, -2, -3, -4

+13 to +16 Excellent
+9 to +12.9 Very Good
+5 to +8.9 Good
+1 to +4.9 Neutral
0 to -4.9 Poor
-5 to -8.9 Very Poor
-9 to -15 Critical

Hydration Scoring Scale

Water Intake (per day)*	Score
≥ 2.0 to 2.5 liters	2
1.5 to 2 liters	1
1 to 1.5 liters	0
0 to 1 liters	-1

Food Scoring Scale

Meal Quality	Score
Meal does not exist	1
Healthy and in reasonable quantity	2
Healthy but in excess	1
Neutral meal	0
Unhealthy meal	-1
Unhealthy and in excess	-2
Includes ice cream, cakes, soft drinks, or French fries	-1 per item

Physical Activity Scoring Scale

Activity Type	Score
Walking – 15 minutes	1
Running – 10 minutes	1
Other intense activities – 10 minutes	1
Sitting – every 2 hours continuously	-1

| Date / / | Week 8 |

Daily Score

| Water Intake | + | Break fast | Morning snack | Lunch | Afternoon snack | Dinner | + | Physical Activity | = | |

Water Intake	Break fast	Morning snack	Lunch	Afternoon snack	Dinner	Physical Activity
2	2	2	2	2	2	4
1	1	1	1	1	1	3
0	0	0	0	0	0	2
-1	-1	-1	-1	-1	-1	1
	-2	-2	-2	-2	-2	0
						-1
						-2
						-3
						-4

+13 to +16 Excellent
+9 to +12.9 Very Good
+5 to +8.9 Good
+1 to +4.9 Neutral
0 to -4.9 Poor
-5 to -8.9 Very Poor
-9 to -15 Critical

Hydration Scoring Scale

Water Intake (per day)*	Score
≥ 2.0 to 2.5 liters	2
1.5 to 2 liters	1
1 to 1.5 liters	0
0 to 1 liters	-1

Food Scoring Scale

Meal Quality	Score
Meal does not exist	1
Healthy and in reasonable quantity	2
Healthy but in excess	1
Neutral meal	0
Unhealthy meal	-1
Unhealthy and in excess	-2
Includes ice cream, cakes, soft drinks, or French fries	-1 per item

Physical Activity Scoring Scale

Activity Type	Score
Walking – 15 minutes	1
Running – 10 minutes	1
Other intense activities – 10 minutes	1
Sitting – every 2 hours continuously	-1

Daily Score

Water Intake + Break fast — Morning snack — Lunch — Afternoon snack — Dinner + Physical Activity = ( )

Water Intake	Break fast	Morning snack	Lunch	Afternoon snack	Dinner	Physical Activity
2	2	2	2	2	2	4
1	1	1	1	1	1	3
0	0	0	0	0	0	2
-1	-1	-1	-1	-1	-1	1
	-2	-2	-2	-2	-2	0
						-1
						-2
						-3
						-4

+13 to +16 Excellent
+9 to +12.9 Very Good
+5 to +8.9 Good
+1 to +4.9 Neutral
0 to -4.9 Poor
-5 to -8.9 Very Poor
-9 to -15 Critical

Hydration Scoring Scale

Water Intake (per day)*	Score
≥ 2.0 to 2.5 liters	2
1.5 to 2 liters	1
1 to 1.5 liters	0
0 to 1 liters	-1

Food Scoring Scale

Meal Quality	Score
Meal does not exist	1
Healthy and in reasonable quantity	2
Healthy but in excess	1
Neutral meal	0
Unhealthy meal	-1
Unhealthy and in excess	-2
Includes ice cream, cakes, soft drinks, or French fries	-1 per item

Physical Activity Scoring Scale

Activity Type	Score
Walking – 15 minutes	1
Running – 10 minutes	1
Other intense activities – 10 minutes	1
Sitting – every 2 hours continuously	-1

Daily Score

(Water Intake) + (Break fast) (Morning snack) (Lunch) (Afternoon snack) (Dinner) + (Physical Activity) = ( )

Water Intake	Break fast	Morning snack	Lunch	Afternoon snack	Dinner	Physical Activity
2	2	2	2	2	2	4
1	1	1	1	1	1	3
0	0	0	0	0	0	2
-1	-1	-1	-1	-1	-1	1
	-2	-2	-2	-2	-2	0
						-1
						-2
						-3
						-4

+13 to +16 Excellent
+9 to +12.9 Very Good
+5 to +8.9 Good
+1 to +4.9 Neutral
0 to -4.9 Poor
-5 to -8.9 Very Poor
-9 to -15 Critical

Hydration Scoring Scale

Water Intake (per day)*	Score
≥ 2.0 to 2.5 liters	2
1.5 to 2 liters	1
1 to 1.5 liters	0
0 to 1 liters	-1

Food Scoring Scale

Meal Quality	Score
Meal does not exist	1
Healthy and in reasonable quantity	2
Healthy but in excess	1
Neutral meal	0
Unhealthy meal	-1
Unhealthy and in excess	-2
Includes ice cream, cakes, soft drinks, or French fries	-1 per item

Physical Activity Scoring Scale

Activity Type	Score
Walking – 15 minutes	1
Running – 10 minutes	1
Other intense activities – 10 minutes	1
Sitting – every 2 hours continuously	-1

Water Intake	+	Break fast	Morning snack	Lunch	Afternoon snack	Dinner	+	Physical Activity	=	Daily Score

Water Intake: 2, 1, 0, -1

Break fast: 2, 1, 0, -1, -2

Morning snack: 2, 1, 0, -1, -2

Lunch: 2, 1, 0, -1, -2

Afternoon snack: 2, 1, 0, -1, -2

Dinner: 2, 1, 0, -1, -2

Physical Activity: 4, 3, 2, 1, 0, -1, -2, -3, -4

+13 to +16 Excellent
+9 to +12.9 Very Good
+5 to +8.9 Good
+1 to +4.9 Neutral
0 to -4.9 Poor
-5 to -8.9 Very Poor
-9 to -15 Critical

Hydration Scoring Scale

Water Intake (per day)*	Score
≥ 2.0 to 2.5 liters	2
1.5 to 2 liters	1
1 to 1.5 liters	0
0 to 1 liters	-1

Food Scoring Scale

Meal Quality	Score
Meal does not exist	1
Healthy and in reasonable quantity	2
Healthy but in excess	1
Neutral meal	0
Unhealthy meal	-1
Unhealthy and in excess	-2
Includes ice cream, cakes, soft drinks, or French fries	-1 per item

Physical Activity Scoring Scale

Activity Type	Score
Walking – 15 minutes	1
Running – 10 minutes	1
Other intense activities – 10 minutes	1
Sitting – every 2 hours continuously	-1

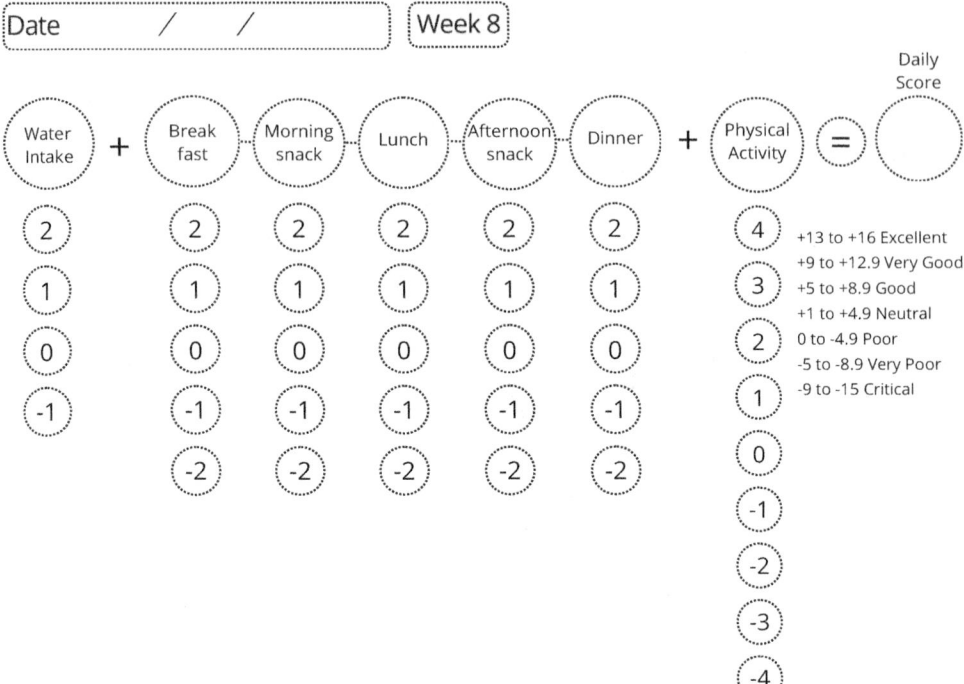

Date ___ / ___ / ___   Week 8

Water Intake + Break fast Morning snack Lunch Afternoon snack Dinner + Physical Activity = Daily Score

Water Intake	Breakfast	Morning snack	Lunch	Afternoon snack	Dinner	Physical Activity
2	2	2	2	2	2	4
1	1	1	1	1	1	3
0	0	0	0	0	0	2
-1	-1	-1	-1	-1	-1	1
	-2	-2	-2	-2	-2	0
						-1
						-2
						-3
						-4

+13 to +16 Excellent
+9 to +12.9 Very Good
+5 to +8.9 Good
+1 to +4.9 Neutral
0 to -4.9 Poor
-5 to -8.9 Very Poor
-9 to -15 Critical

Hydration Scoring Scale

Water Intake (per day)*	Score
≥ 2.0 to 2.5 liters	2
1.5 to 2 liters	1
1 to 1.5 liters	0
0 to 1 liters	-1

Food Scoring Scale

Meal Quality	Score
Meal does not exist	1
Healthy and in reasonable quantity	2
Healthy but in excess	1
Neutral meal	0
Unhealthy meal	-1
Unhealthy and in excess	-2
Includes ice cream, cakes, soft drinks, or French fries	-1 per item

Physical Activity Scoring Scale

Activity Type	Score
Walking – 15 minutes	1
Running – 10 minutes	1
Other intense activities – 10 minutes	1
Sitting – every 2 hours continuously	-1

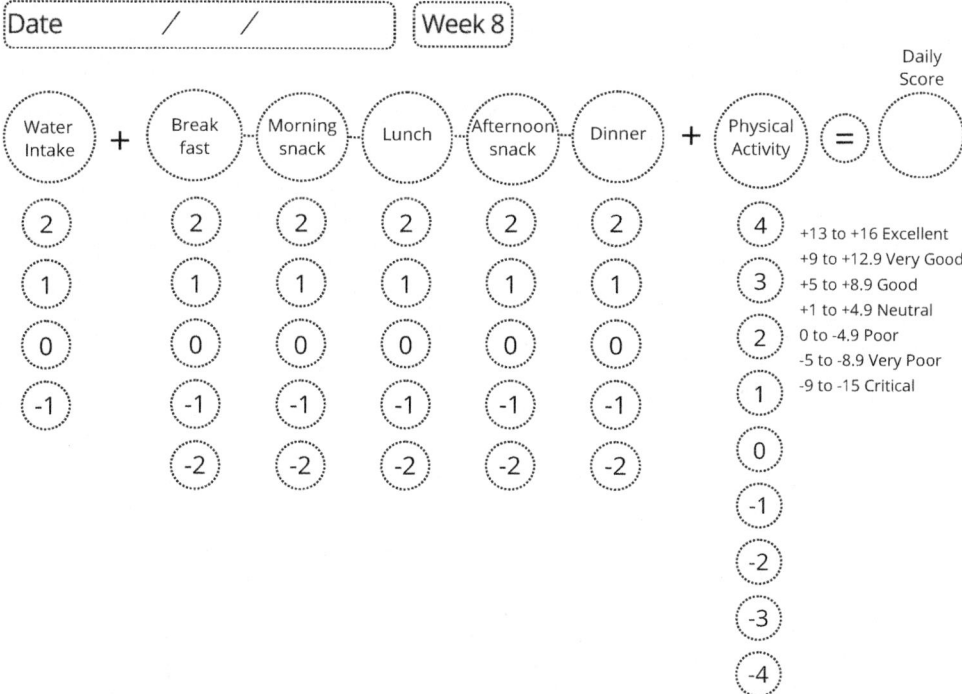

End of Week 8 – Weekly Summary

Two months in — your consistency is building momentum. Trust the process, and keep showing up.

Date _____ / ____ / ____   Week 9

Daily Score

(Water Intake) + (Break fast) (Morning snack) (Lunch) (Afternoon snack) (Dinner) + (Physical Activity) = ( )

Water Intake	Breakfast	Morning snack	Lunch	Afternoon snack	Dinner	Physical Activity
2	2	2	2	2	2	4
1	1	1	1	1	1	3
0	0	0	0	0	0	2
-1	-1	-1	-1	-1	-1	1
	-2	-2	-2	-2	-2	0
						-1
						-2
						-3
						-4

+13 to +16 Excellent
+9 to +12.9 Very Good
+5 to +8.9 Good
+1 to +4.9 Neutral
0 to -4.9 Poor
-5 to -8.9 Very Poor
-9 to -15 Critical

Hydration Scoring Scale

Water Intake (per day)*	Score
≥ 2.0 to 2.5 liters	2
1.5 to 2 liters	1
1 to 1.5 liters	0
0 to 1 liters	-1

Food Scoring Scale

Meal Quality	Score
Meal does not exist	1
Healthy and in reasonable quantity	2
Healthy but in excess	1
Neutral meal	0
Unhealthy meal	-1
Unhealthy and in excess	-2
Includes ice cream, cakes, soft drinks, or French fries	-1 per item

Physical Activity Scoring Scale

Activity Type	Score
Walking – 15 minutes	1
Running – 10 minutes	1
Other intense activities – 10 minutes	1
Sitting – every 2 hours continuously	-1

Daily Score

Water Intake + Break fast   Morning snack   Lunch   Afternoon snack   Dinner + Physical Activity = ( )

Water Intake	Break fast	Morning snack	Lunch	Afternoon snack	Dinner	Physical Activity
2	2	2	2	2	2	4
1	1	1	1	1	1	3
0	0	0	0	0	0	2
-1	-1	-1	-1	-1	-1	1
	-2	-2	-2	-2	-2	0
						-1
						-2
						-3
						-4

+13 to +16 Excellent
+9 to +12.9 Very Good
+5 to +8.9 Good
+1 to +4.9 Neutral
0 to -4.9 Poor
-5 to -8.9 Very Poor
-9 to -15 Critical

Hydration Scoring Scale

Water Intake (per day)*	Score
≥ 2.0 to 2.5 liters	2
1.5 to 2 liters	1
1 to 1.5 liters	0
0 to 1 liters	-1

Food Scoring Scale

Meal Quality	Score
Meal does not exist	1
Healthy and in reasonable quantity	2
Healthy but in excess	1
Neutral meal	0
Unhealthy meal	-1
Unhealthy and in excess	-2
Includes ice cream, cakes, soft drinks, or French fries	-1 per item

Physical Activity Scoring Scale

Activity Type	Score
Walking – 15 minutes	1
Running – 10 minutes	1
Other intense activities – 10 minutes	1
Sitting – every 2 hours continuously	-1

| Date / / | Week 9 |

Daily Score

(Water Intake) + (Break fast) (Morning snack) (Lunch) (Afternoon snack) (Dinner) + (Physical Activity) = ( )

Water Intake		Breakfast	Morning snack	Lunch	Afternoon snack	Dinner		Physical Activity	
2		2	2	2	2	2		4	+13 to +16 Excellent
1		1	1	1	1	1		3	+9 to +12.9 Very Good
0		0	0	0	0	0		2	+5 to +8.9 Good
-1		-1	-1	-1	-1	-1		1	+1 to +4.9 Neutral
		-2	-2	-2	-2	-2		0	0 to -4.9 Poor
								-1	-5 to -8.9 Very Poor
								-2	-9 to -15 Critical
								-3	
								-4	

Hydration Scoring Scale

Water Intake (per day)*	Score
≥ 2.0 to 2.5 liters	2
1.5 to 2 liters	1
1 to 1.5 liters	0
0 to 1 liters	-1

Food Scoring Scale

Meal Quality	Score
Meal does not exist	1
Healthy and in reasonable quantity	2
Healthy but in excess	1
Neutral meal	0
Unhealthy meal	-1
Unhealthy and in excess	-2
Includes ice cream, cakes, soft drinks, or French fries	-1 per item

Physical Activity Scoring Scale

Activity Type	Score
Walking – 15 minutes	1
Running – 10 minutes	1
Other intense activities – 10 minutes	1
Sitting – every 2 hours continuously	-1

Date / /	Week 9

Water Intake + Break fast ⋯ Morning snack ⋯ Lunch ⋯ Afternoon snack ⋯ Dinner + Physical Activity = Daily Score

Water Intake		Break fast	Morning snack	Lunch	Afternoon snack	Dinner		Physical Activity	
2		2	2	2	2	2		4	+13 to +16 Excellent
1		1	1	1	1	1		3	+9 to +12.9 Very Good
0		0	0	0	0	0		2	+5 to +8.9 Good
-1		-1	-1	-1	-1	-1		1	+1 to +4.9 Neutral
		-2	-2	-2	-2	-2		0	0 to -4.9 Poor
								-1	-5 to -8.9 Very Poor
								-2	-9 to -15 Critical
								-3	
								-4	

Hydration Scoring Scale

Water Intake (per day)*	Score
≥ 2.0 to 2.5 liters	2
1.5 to 2 liters	1
1 to 1.5 liters	0
0 to 1 liters	-1

Food Scoring Scale

Meal Quality	Score
Meal does not exist	1
Healthy and in reasonable quantity	2
Healthy but in excess	1
Neutral meal	0
Unhealthy meal	-1
Unhealthy and in excess	-2
Includes ice cream, cakes, soft drinks, or French fries	-1 per item

Physical Activity Scoring Scale

Activity Type	Score
Walking – 15 minutes	1
Running – 10 minutes	1
Other intense activities – 10 minutes	1
Sitting – every 2 hours continuously	-1

| Date | / | / | | Week 9 |

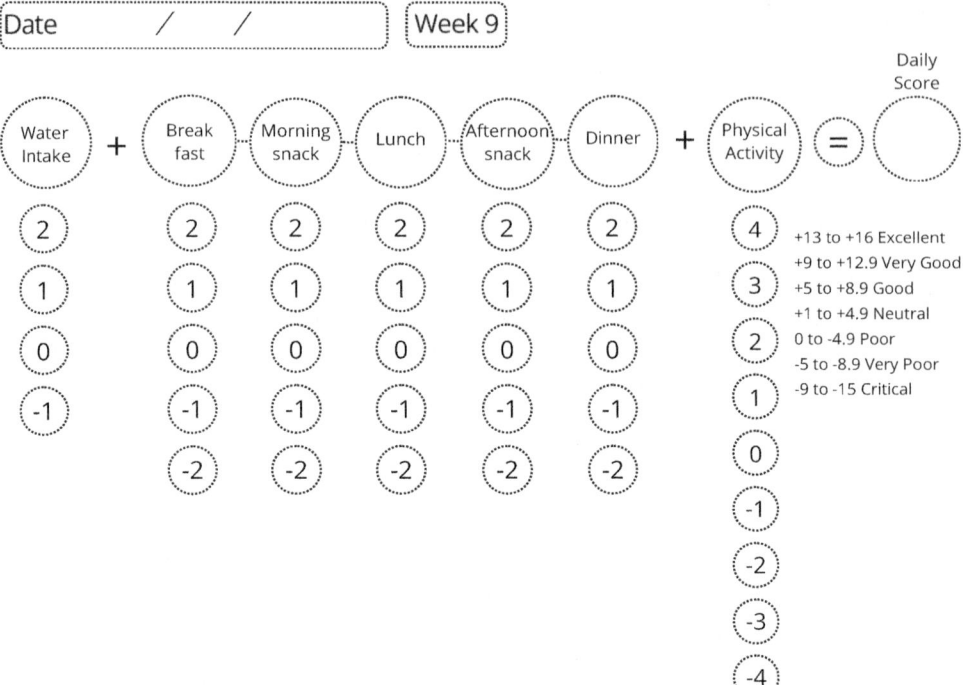

Daily Score

Water Intake + Break fast · Morning snack · Lunch · Afternoon snack · Dinner + Physical Activity = ◯

Water Intake	Break fast	Morning snack	Lunch	Afternoon snack	Dinner	Physical Activity
2	2	2	2	2	2	4
1	1	1	1	1	1	3
0	0	0	0	0	0	2
-1	-1	-1	-1	-1	-1	1
	-2	-2	-2	-2	-2	0
						-1
						-2
						-3
						-4

+13 to +16 Excellent
+9 to +12.9 Very Good
+5 to +8.9 Good
+1 to +4.9 Neutral
0 to -4.9 Poor
-5 to -8.9 Very Poor
-9 to -15 Critical

Hydration Scoring Scale

Water Intake (per day)*	Score
≥ 2.0 to 2.5 liters	2
1.5 to 2 liters	1
1 to 1.5 liters	0
0 to 1 liters	-1

Food Scoring Scale

Meal Quality	Score
Meal does not exist	1
Healthy and in reasonable quantity	2
Healthy but in excess	1
Neutral meal	0
Unhealthy meal	-1
Unhealthy and in excess	-2
Includes ice cream, cakes, soft drinks, or French fries	-1 per item

Physical Activity Scoring Scale

Activity Type	Score
Walking – 15 minutes	1
Running – 10 minutes	1
Other intense activities – 10 minutes	1
Sitting – every 2 hours continuously	-1

Date	/	/		Week 9

Daily Score

Water Intake + Break fast ○ Morning snack ○ Lunch ○ Afternoon snack ○ Dinner + Physical Activity = ○

Water Intake	Break fast	Morning snack	Lunch	Afternoon snack	Dinner	Physical Activity
2	2	2	2	2	2	4
1	1	1	1	1	1	3
0	0	0	0	0	0	2
-1	-1	-1	-1	-1	-1	1
	-2	-2	-2	-2	-2	0
						-1
						-2
						-3
						-4

+13 to +16 Excellent
+9 to +12.9 Very Good
+5 to +8.9 Good
+1 to +4.9 Neutral
0 to -4.9 Poor
-5 to -8.9 Very Poor
-9 to -15 Critical

Hydration Scoring Scale

Water Intake (per day)*	Score
≥ 2.0 to 2.5 liters	2
1.5 to 2 liters	1
1 to 1.5 liters	0
0 to 1 liters	-1

Food Scoring Scale

Meal Quality	Score
Meal does not exist	1
Healthy and in reasonable quantity	2
Healthy but in excess	1
Neutral meal	0
Unhealthy meal	-1
Unhealthy and in excess	-2
Includes ice cream, cakes, soft drinks, or French fries	-1 per item

Physical Activity Scoring Scale

Activity Type	Score
Walking – 15 minutes	1
Running – 10 minutes	1
Other intense activities – 10 minutes	1
Sitting – every 2 hours continuously	-1

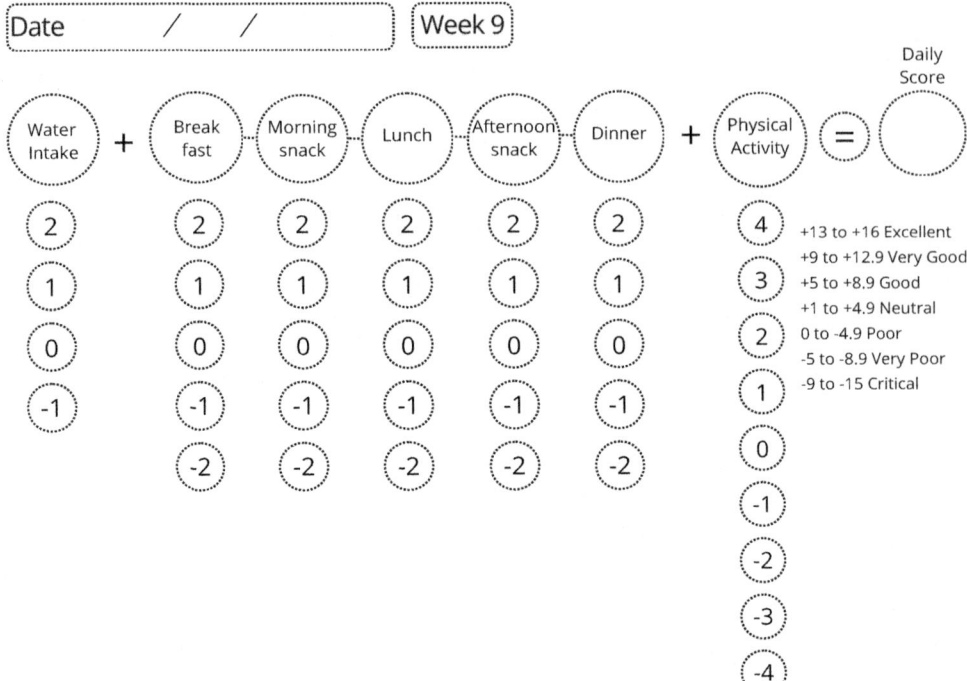

End of Week 9 – Weekly Summary

You've come this far for a reason. Let every small step remind you that lasting change is built one day at a time.

Date _____ / _____ / _____   Week 10

Water Intake + Break fast Morning snack Lunch Afternoon snack Dinner + Physical Activity = Daily Score

Water Intake	Breakfast	Morning snack	Lunch	Afternoon snack	Dinner	Physical Activity	
2	2	2	2	2	2	4	+13 to +16 Excellent
1	1	1	1	1	1	3	+9 to +12.9 Very Good
0	0	0	0	0	0	2	+5 to +8.9 Good
-1	-1	-1	-1	-1	-1	1	+1 to +4.9 Neutral
	-2	-2	-2	-2	-2	0	0 to -4.9 Poor
						-1	-5 to -8.9 Very Poor
						-2	-9 to -15 Critical
						-3	
						-4	

Hydration Scoring Scale

Water Intake (per day)*	Score
≥ 2.0 to 2.5 liters	2
1.5 to 2 liters	1
1 to 1.5 liters	0
0 to 1 liters	-1

Food Scoring Scale

Meal Quality	Score
Meal does not exist	1
Healthy and in reasonable quantity	2
Healthy but in excess	1
Neutral meal	0
Unhealthy meal	-1
Unhealthy and in excess	-2
Includes ice cream, cakes, soft drinks, or French fries	-1 per item

Physical Activity Scoring Scale

Activity Type	Score
Walking – 15 minutes	1
Running – 10 minutes	1
Other intense activities – 10 minutes	1
Sitting – every 2 hours continuously	-1

Date	/	/		Week 10

Daily Score

(Water Intake) + (Break fast) (Morning snack) (Lunch) (Afternoon snack) (Dinner) + (Physical Activity) = ( )

Water Intake	Break fast	Morning snack	Lunch	Afternoon snack	Dinner	Physical Activity	
2	2	2	2	2	2	4	+13 to +16 Excellent
1	1	1	1	1	1	3	+9 to +12.9 Very Good
0	0	0	0	0	0	2	+5 to +8.9 Good
-1	-1	-1	-1	-1	-1	1	+1 to +4.9 Neutral
	-2	-2	-2	-2	-2	0	0 to -4.9 Poor
						-1	-5 to -8.9 Very Poor
						-2	-9 to -15 Critical
						-3	
						-4	

Hydration Scoring Scale

Water Intake (per day)*	Score
≥ 2.0 to 2.5 liters	2
1.5 to 2 liters	1
1 to 1.5 liters	0
0 to 1 liters	-1

Food Scoring Scale

Meal Quality	Score
Meal does not exist	1
Healthy and in reasonable quantity	2
Healthy but in excess	1
Neutral meal	0
Unhealthy meal	-1
Unhealthy and in excess	-2
Includes ice cream, cakes, soft drinks, or French fries	-1 per item

Physical Activity Scoring Scale

Activity Type	Score
Walking – 15 minutes	1
Running – 10 minutes	1
Other intense activities – 10 minutes	1
Sitting – every 2 hours continuously	-1

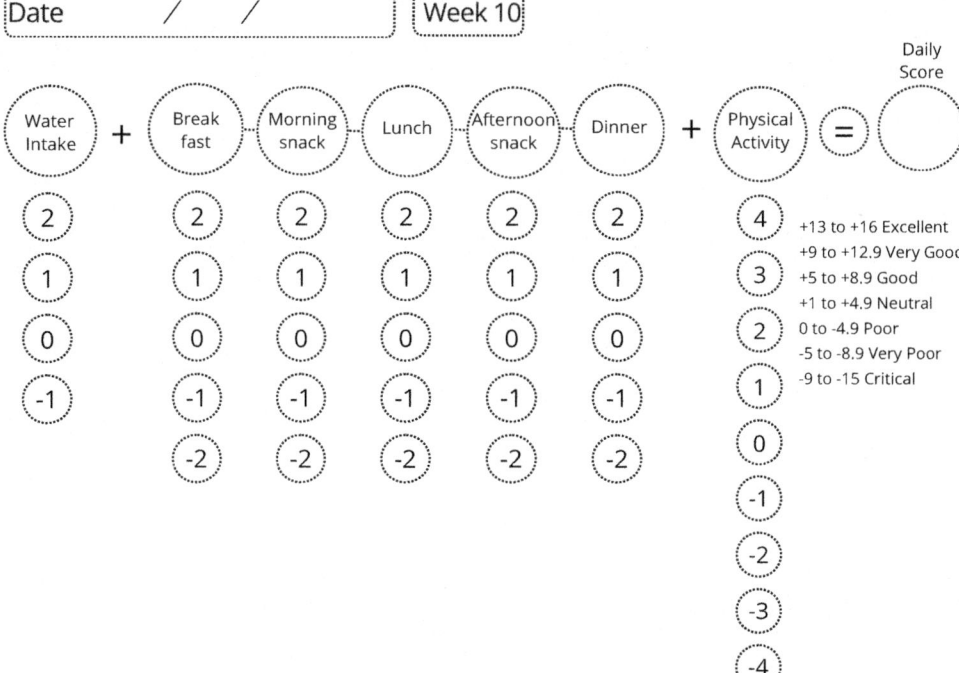

Hydration Scoring Scale	
Water Intake (per day)*	**Score**
≥ 2.0 to 2.5 liters	2
1.5 to 2 liters	1
1 to 1.5 liters	0
0 to 1 liters	-1

Food Scoring Scale	
Meal Quality	**Score**
Meal does not exist	1
Healthy and in reasonable quantity	2
Healthy but in excess	1
Neutral meal	0
Unhealthy meal	-1
Unhealthy and in excess	-2
Includes ice cream, cakes, soft drinks, or French fries	-1 per item

Physical Activity Scoring Scale	
Activity Type	**Score**
Walking – 15 minutes	1
Running – 10 minutes	1
Other intense activities – 10 minutes	1
Sitting – every 2 hours continuously	-1

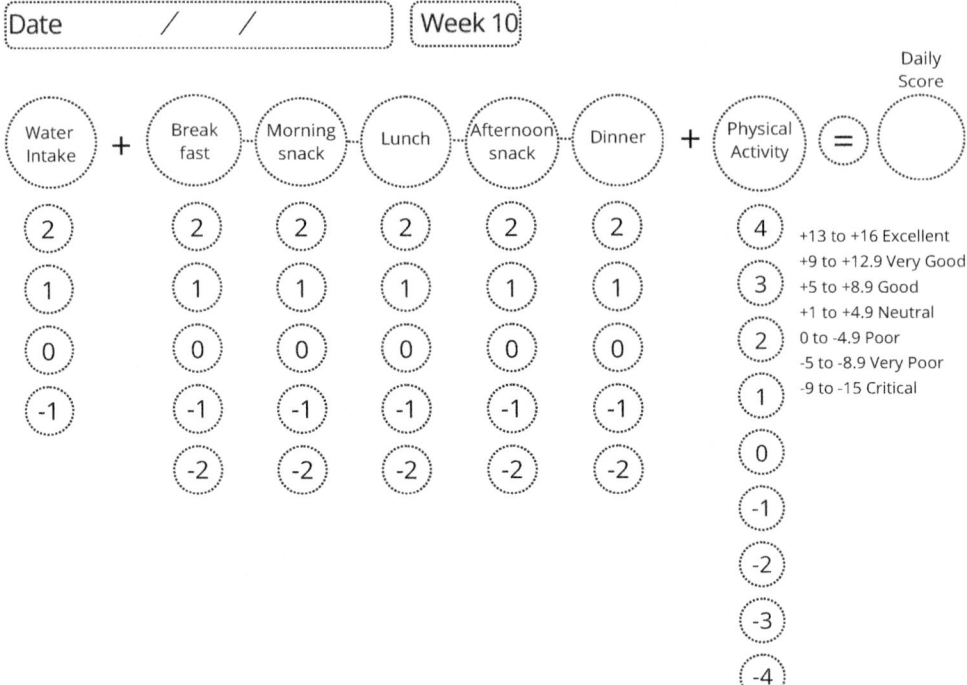

Daily Score

Water Intake + Break fast — Morning snack — Lunch — Afternoon snack — Dinner + Physical Activity = ○

+13 to +16 Excellent
+9 to +12.9 Very Good
+5 to +8.9 Good
+1 to +4.9 Neutral
0 to -4.9 Poor
-5 to -8.9 Very Poor
-9 to -15 Critical

Hydration Scoring Scale

Water Intake (per day)*	Score
≥ 2.0 to 2.5 liters	2
1.5 to 2 liters	1
1 to 1.5 liters	0
0 to 1 liters	-1

Food Scoring Scale

Meal Quality	Score
Meal does not exist	1
Healthy and in reasonable quantity	2
Healthy but in excess	1
Neutral meal	0
Unhealthy meal	-1
Unhealthy and in excess	-2
Includes ice cream, cakes, soft drinks, or French fries	-1 per item

Physical Activity Scoring Scale

Activity Type	Score
Walking – 15 minutes	1
Running – 10 minutes	1
Other intense activities – 10 minutes	1
Sitting – every 2 hours continuously	-1

Date   /   /   Week 10

Daily Score

(Water Intake) + (Break fast) (Morning snack) (Lunch) (Afternoon snack) (Dinner) + (Physical Activity) = ( )

Water Intake / Breakfast / Morning snack / Lunch / Afternoon snack / Dinner:
- 2
- 1
- 0
- -1
- -2 (except Water Intake, which stops at -1)

Physical Activity:
- 4
- 3
- 2
- 1
- 0
- -1
- -2
- -3
- -4

+13 to +16 Excellent
+9 to +12.9 Very Good
+5 to +8.9 Good
+1 to +4.9 Neutral
0 to -4.9 Poor
-5 to -8.9 Very Poor
-9 to -15 Critical

Hydration Scoring Scale

Water Intake (per day)*	Score
≥ 2.0 to 2.5 liters	2
1.5 to 2 liters	1
1 to 1.5 liters	0
0 to 1 liters	-1

Food Scoring Scale

Meal Quality	Score
Meal does not exist	1
Healthy and in reasonable quantity	2
Healthy but in excess	1
Neutral meal	0
Unhealthy meal	-1
Unhealthy and in excess	-2
Includes ice cream, cakes, soft drinks, or French fries	-1 per item

Physical Activity Scoring Scale

Activity Type	Score
Walking – 15 minutes	1
Running – 10 minutes	1
Other intense activities – 10 minutes	1
Sitting – every 2 hours continuously	-1

Date   /   /   Week 10

Daily Score

(Water Intake) + (Breakfast) (Morning snack) (Lunch) (Afternoon snack) (Dinner) + (Physical Activity) = ( )

Water Intake	Breakfast	Morning snack	Lunch	Afternoon snack	Dinner	Physical Activity	
2	2	2	2	2	2	4	+13 to +16 Excellent
1	1	1	1	1	1	3	+9 to +12.9 Very Good
0	0	0	0	0	0	2	+5 to +8.9 Good
-1	-1	-1	-1	-1	-1	1	+1 to +4.9 Neutral
	-2	-2	-2	-2	-2	0	0 to -4.9 Poor
						-1	-5 to -8.9 Very Poor
						-2	-9 to -15 Critical
						-3	
						-4	

Hydration Scoring Scale

Water Intake (per day)*	Score
≥ 2.0 to 2.5 liters	2
1.5 to 2 liters	1
1 to 1.5 liters	0
0 to 1 liters	-1

Food Scoring Scale

Meal Quality	Score
Meal does not exist	1
Healthy and in reasonable quantity	2
Healthy but in excess	1
Neutral meal	0
Unhealthy meal	-1
Unhealthy and in excess	-2
Includes ice cream, cakes, soft drinks, or French fries	-1 per item

Physical Activity Scoring Scale

Activity Type	Score
Walking – 15 minutes	1
Running – 10 minutes	1
Other intense activities – 10 minutes	1
Sitting – every 2 hours continuously	-1

96

Date / /	Week 10

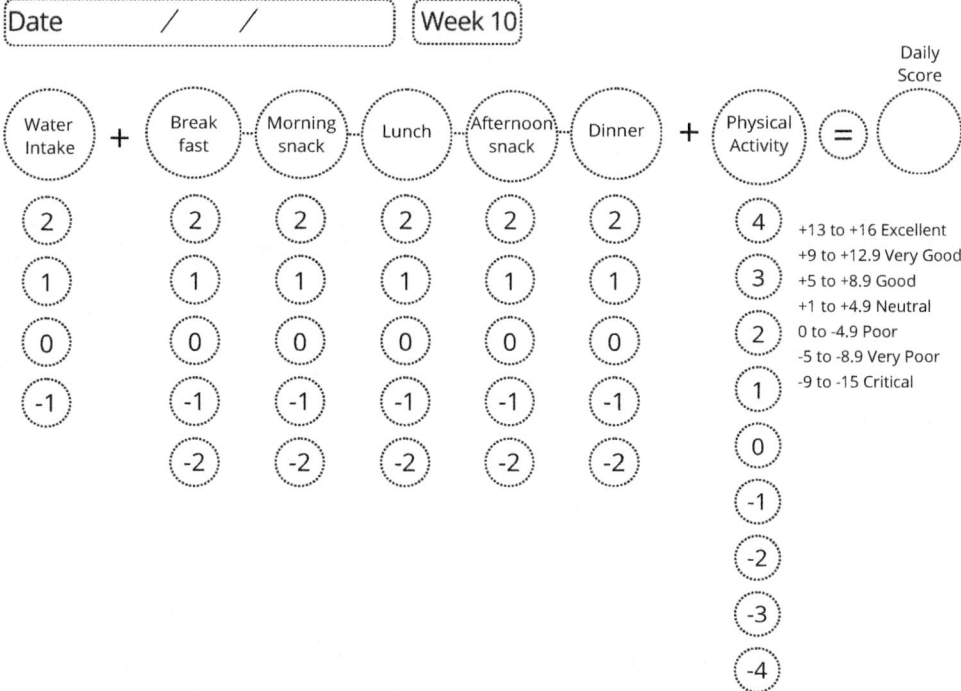

End of Week 10 – Weekly Summary

Ten weeks in — your commitment is turning into transformation. Stay focused, you're building something real and lasting.

Daily
Score

Water Intake + Break fast   Morning snack   Lunch   Afternoon snack   Dinner + Physical Activity = ( )

| Water Intake | | Break fast | Morning snack | Lunch | Afternoon snack | Dinner | | Physical Activity | |

2   2   2   2   2   2   4   +13 to +16 Excellent

1   1   1   1   1   1   3   +9 to +12.9 Very Good

0   0   0   0   0   0   2   +5 to +8.9 Good

-1   -1   -1   -1   -1   -1   1   +1 to +4.9 Neutral

          -2   -2   -2   -2   -2   0   0 to -4.9 Poor

                                     -1   -5 to -8.9 Very Poor

                                     -2   -9 to -15 Critical

                                     -3

                                     -4

Hydration Scoring Scale

Water Intake (per day)*	Score
≥ 2.0 to 2.5 liters	2
1.5 to 2 liters	1
1 to 1.5 liters	0
0 to 1 liters	-1

Food Scoring Scale

Meal Quality	Score
Meal does not exist	1
Healthy and in reasonable quantity	2
Healthy but in excess	1
Neutral meal	0
Unhealthy meal	-1
Unhealthy and in excess	-2
Includes ice cream, cakes, soft drinks, or French fries	-1 per item

Physical Activity Scoring Scale

Activity Type	Score
Walking – 15 minutes	1
Running – 10 minutes	1
Other intense activities – 10 minutes	1
Sitting – every 2 hours continuously	-1

Date	/	/		Week 11

Daily Score

Water Intake + Break fast — Morning snack — Lunch — Afternoon snack — Dinner + Physical Activity = ( )

Water Intake	Break fast	Morning snack	Lunch	Afternoon snack	Dinner	Physical Activity	
2	2	2	2	2	2	4	+13 to +16 Excellent
1	1	1	1	1	1	3	+9 to +12.9 Very Good
0	0	0	0	0	0	2	+5 to +8.9 Good
-1	-1	-1	-1	-1	-1	1	+1 to +4.9 Neutral
	-2	-2	-2	-2	-2	0	0 to -4.9 Poor
						-1	-5 to -8.9 Very Poor
						-2	-9 to -15 Critical
						-3	
						-4	

Hydration Scoring Scale

Water Intake (per day)*	Score
≥ 2.0 to 2.5 liters	2
1.5 to 2 liters	1
1 to 1.5 liters	0
0 to 1 liters	-1

Food Scoring Scale

Meal Quality	Score
Meal does not exist	1
Healthy and in reasonable quantity	2
Healthy but in excess	1
Neutral meal	0
Unhealthy meal	-1
Unhealthy and in excess	-2
Includes ice cream, cakes, soft drinks, or French fries	-1 per item

Physical Activity Scoring Scale

Activity Type	Score
Walking – 15 minutes	1
Running – 10 minutes	1
Other intense activities – 10 minutes	1
Sitting – every 2 hours continuously	-1

Daily Score

Water Intake + Break fast | Morning snack | Lunch | Afternoon snack | Dinner + Physical Activity = ( )

Water Intake		Break fast	Morning snack	Lunch	Afternoon snack	Dinner		Physical Activity
2	+	2	2	2	2	2	+	4
1		1	1	1	1	1		3
0		0	0	0	0	0		2
-1		-1	-1	-1	-1	-1		1
		-2	-2	-2	-2	-2		0
								-1
								-2
								-3
								-4

+13 to +16 Excellent
+9 to +12.9 Very Good
+5 to +8.9 Good
+1 to +4.9 Neutral
0 to -4.9 Poor
-5 to -8.9 Very Poor
-9 to -15 Critical

Hydration Scoring Scale

Water Intake (per day)*	Score
≥ 2.0 to 2.5 liters	2
1.5 to 2 liters	1
1 to 1.5 liters	0
0 to 1 liters	-1

Food Scoring Scale

Meal Quality	Score
Meal does not exist	1
Healthy and in reasonable quantity	2
Healthy but in excess	1
Neutral meal	0
Unhealthy meal	-1
Unhealthy and in excess	-2
Includes ice cream, cakes, soft drinks, or French fries	-1 per item

Physical Activity Scoring Scale

Activity Type	Score
Walking – 15 minutes	1
Running – 10 minutes	1
Other intense activities – 10 minutes	1
Sitting – every 2 hours continuously	-1

Date / /	Week 11

Daily Score

Water Intake + Break fast | Morning snack | Lunch | Afternoon snack | Dinner + Physical Activity = ( )

Water Intake	Break fast	Morning snack	Lunch	Afternoon snack	Dinner	Physical Activity
2	2	2	2	2	2	4
1	1	1	1	1	1	3
0	0	0	0	0	0	2
-1	-1	-1	-1	-1	-1	1
	-2	-2	-2	-2	-2	0
						-1
						-2
						-3
						-4

+13 to +16 Excellent
+9 to +12.9 Very Good
+5 to +8.9 Good
+1 to +4.9 Neutral
0 to -4.9 Poor
-5 to -8.9 Very Poor
-9 to -15 Critical

Hydration Scoring Scale

Water Intake (per day)*	Score
≥ 2.0 to 2.5 liters	2
1.5 to 2 liters	1
1 to 1.5 liters	0
0 to 1 liters	-1

Food Scoring Scale

Meal Quality	Score
Meal does not exist	1
Healthy and in reasonable quantity	2
Healthy but in excess	1
Neutral meal	0
Unhealthy meal	-1
Unhealthy and in excess	-2
Includes ice cream, cakes, soft drinks, or French fries	-1 per item

Physical Activity Scoring Scale

Activity Type	Score
Walking – 15 minutes	1
Running – 10 minutes	1
Other intense activities – 10 minutes	1
Sitting – every 2 hours continuously	-1

Daily Score

Water Intake + Break fast Morning snack Lunch Afternoon snack Dinner + Physical Activity = ( )

Water Intake

2
1
0
-1

Break fast

2
1
0
-1
-2

Morning snack

2
1
0
-1
-2

Lunch

2
1
0
-1
-2

Afternoon snack

2
1
0
-1
-2

Dinner

2
1
0
-1
-2

Physical Activity

4
3
2
1
0
-1
-2
-3
-4

+13 to +16 Excellent
+9 to +12.9 Very Good
+5 to +8.9 Good
+1 to +4.9 Neutral
0 to -4.9 Poor
-5 to -8.9 Very Poor
-9 to -15 Critical

Hydration Scoring Scale

Water Intake (per day)*	Score
≥ 2.0 to 2.5 liters	2
1.5 to 2 liters	1
1 to 1.5 liters	0
0 to 1 liters	-1

Food Scoring Scale

Meal Quality	Score
Meal does not exist	1
Healthy and in reasonable quantity	2
Healthy but in excess	1
Neutral meal	0
Unhealthy meal	-1
Unhealthy and in excess	-2
Includes ice cream, cakes, soft drinks, or French fries	-1 per item

Physical Activity Scoring Scale

Activity Type	Score
Walking – 15 minutes	1
Running – 10 minutes	1
Other intense activities – 10 minutes	1
Sitting – every 2 hours continuously	-1

Water Intake + Break fast + Morning snack + Lunch + Afternoon snack + Dinner + Physical Activity = Daily Score

Water Intake	Break fast	Morning snack	Lunch	Afternoon snack	Dinner	Physical Activity
2	2	2	2	2	2	4
1	1	1	1	1	1	3
0	0	0	0	0	0	2
-1	-1	-1	-1	-1	-1	1
	-2	-2	-2	-2	-2	0
						-1
						-2
						-3
						-4

+13 to +16 Excellent
+9 to +12.9 Very Good
+5 to +8.9 Good
+1 to +4.9 Neutral
0 to -4.9 Poor
-5 to -8.9 Very Poor
-9 to -15 Critical

Hydration Scoring Scale

Water Intake (per day)*	Score
≥ 2.0 to 2.5 liters	2
1.5 to 2 liters	1
1 to 1.5 liters	0
0 to 1 liters	-1

Food Scoring Scale

Meal Quality	Score
Meal does not exist	1
Healthy and in reasonable quantity	2
Healthy but in excess	1
Neutral meal	0
Unhealthy meal	-1
Unhealthy and in excess	-2
Includes ice cream, cakes, soft drinks, or French fries	-1 per item

Physical Activity Scoring Scale

Activity Type	Score
Walking – 15 minutes	1
Running – 10 minutes	1
Other intense activities – 10 minutes	1
Sitting – every 2 hours continuously	-1

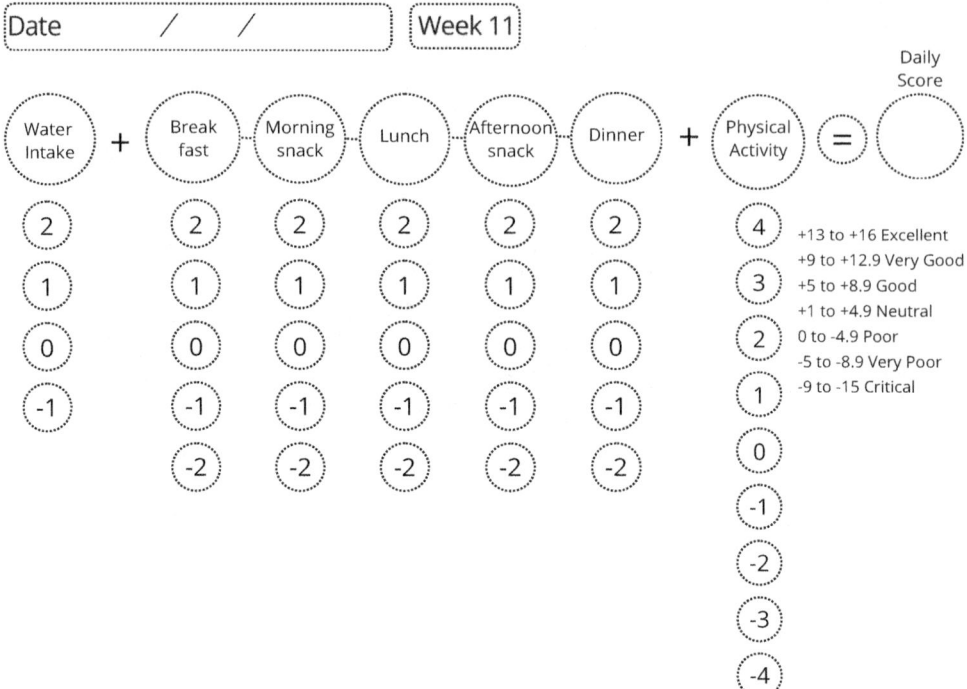

End of Week 11 – Weekly Summary

You've already proven you can stay the course — now is the time to push forward with confidence and pride.

| Date | / | / | | Week 12 |

Daily Score

Water Intake + Break fast | Morning snack | Lunch | Afternoon snack | Dinner + Physical Activity = ( )

Water Intake	Break fast	Morning snack	Lunch	Afternoon snack	Dinner	Physical Activity	
2	2	2	2	2	2	4	+13 to +16 Excellent
1	1	1	1	1	1	3	+9 to +12.9 Very Good
0	0	0	0	0	0	2	+5 to +8.9 Good
-1	-1	-1	-1	-1	-1	1	+1 to +4.9 Neutral
	-2	-2	-2	-2	-2	0	0 to -4.9 Poor
						-1	-5 to -8.9 Very Poor
						-2	-9 to -15 Critical
						-3	
						-4	

Hydration Scoring Scale

Water Intake (per day)*	Score
≥ 2.0 to 2.5 liters	2
1.5 to 2 liters	1
1 to 1.5 liters	0
0 to 1 liters	-1

Food Scoring Scale

Meal Quality	Score
Meal does not exist	1
Healthy and in reasonable quantity	2
Healthy but in excess	1
Neutral meal	0
Unhealthy meal	-1
Unhealthy and in excess	-2
Includes ice cream, cakes, soft drinks, or French fries	-1 per item

Physical Activity Scoring Scale

Activity Type	Score
Walking – 15 minutes	1
Running – 10 minutes	1
Other intense activities – 10 minutes	1
Sitting – every 2 hours continuously	-1

Daily Score

Water Intake	+	Break fast	Morning snack	Lunch	Afternoon snack	Dinner	+	Physical Activity	=	( )

Water Intake: 2, 1, 0, -1

Break fast: 2, 1, 0, -1, -2

Morning snack: 2, 1, 0, -1, -2

Lunch: 2, 1, 0, -1, -2

Afternoon snack: 2, 1, 0, -1, -2

Dinner: 2, 1, 0, -1, -2

Physical Activity: 4, 3, 2, 1, 0, -1, -2, -3, -4

+13 to +16 Excellent
+9 to +12.9 Very Good
+5 to +8.9 Good
+1 to +4.9 Neutral
0 to -4.9 Poor
-5 to -8.9 Very Poor
-9 to -15 Critical

Hydration Scoring Scale

Water Intake (per day)*	Score
≥ 2.0 to 2.5 liters	2
1.5 to 2 liters	1
1 to 1.5 liters	0
0 to 1 liters	-1

Food Scoring Scale

Meal Quality	Score
Meal does not exist	1
Healthy and in reasonable quantity	2
Healthy but in excess	1
Neutral meal	0
Unhealthy meal	-1
Unhealthy and in excess	-2
Includes ice cream, cakes, soft drinks, or French fries	-1 per item

Physical Activity Scoring Scale

Activity Type	Score
Walking – 15 minutes	1
Running – 10 minutes	1
Other intense activities – 10 minutes	1
Sitting – every 2 hours continuously	-1

Water Intake + Break fast ∘ Morning snack ∘ Lunch ∘ Afternoon snack ∘ Dinner + Physical Activity = Daily Score

Water Intake	Break fast	Morning snack	Lunch	Afternoon snack	Dinner	Physical Activity
2	2	2	2	2	2	4
1	1	1	1	1	1	3
0	0	0	0	0	0	2
-1	-1	-1	-1	-1	-1	1
	-2	-2	-2	-2	-2	0
						-1
						-2
						-3
						-4

+13 to +16 Excellent
+9 to +12.9 Very Good
+5 to +8.9 Good
+1 to +4.9 Neutral
0 to -4.9 Poor
-5 to -8.9 Very Poor
-9 to -15 Critical

Hydration Scoring Scale

Water Intake (per day)*	Score
≥ 2.0 to 2.5 liters	2
1.5 to 2 liters	1
1 to 1.5 liters	0
0 to 1 liters	-1

Food Scoring Scale

Meal Quality	Score
Meal does not exist	1
Healthy and in reasonable quantity	2
Healthy but in excess	1
Neutral meal	0
Unhealthy meal	-1
Unhealthy and in excess	-2
Includes ice cream, cakes, soft drinks, or French fries	-1 per item

Physical Activity Scoring Scale

Activity Type	Score
Walking – 15 minutes	1
Running – 10 minutes	1
Other intense activities – 10 minutes	1
Sitting – every 2 hours continuously	-1

Daily Score

(Water Intake) + (Break fast) (Morning snack) (Lunch) (Afternoon snack) (Dinner) + (Physical Activity) (=) ( )

Water Intake	Break fast	Morning snack	Lunch	Afternoon snack	Dinner	Physical Activity
2	2	2	2	2	2	4
1	1	1	1	1	1	3
0	0	0	0	0	0	2
-1	-1	-1	-1	-1	-1	1
	-2	-2	-2	-2	-2	0
						-1
						-2
						-3
						-4

+13 to +16 Excellent
+9 to +12.9 Very Good
+5 to +8.9 Good
+1 to +4.9 Neutral
0 to -4.9 Poor
-5 to -8.9 Very Poor
-9 to -15 Critical

Hydration Scoring Scale

Water Intake (per day)*	Score
≥ 2.0 to 2.5 liters	2
1.5 to 2 liters	1
1 to 1.5 liters	0
0 to 1 liters	-1

Food Scoring Scale

Meal Quality	Score
Meal does not exist	1
Healthy and in reasonable quantity	2
Healthy but in excess	1
Neutral meal	0
Unhealthy meal	-1
Unhealthy and in excess	-2
Includes ice cream, cakes, soft drinks, or French fries	-1 per item

Physical Activity Scoring Scale

Activity Type	Score
Walking – 15 minutes	1
Running – 10 minutes	1
Other intense activities – 10 minutes	1
Sitting – every 2 hours continuously	-1

Water Intake	+	Break fast	Morning snack	Lunch	Afternoon snack	Dinner	+	Physical Activity	=	Daily Score

Water Intake / Breakfast / Morning snack / Lunch / Afternoon snack / Dinner options:

- 2
- 1
- 0
- -1
- -2 (Breakfast, Morning snack, Lunch, Afternoon snack, Dinner)

Physical Activity options: 4, 3, 2, 1, 0, -1, -2, -3, -4

Daily Score scale:

+13 to +16 Excellent
+9 to +12.9 Very Good
+5 to +8.9 Good
+1 to +4.9 Neutral
0 to -4.9 Poor
-5 to -8.9 Very Poor
-9 to -15 Critical

Hydration Scoring Scale

Water Intake (per day)*	Score
≥ 2.0 to 2.5 liters	2
1.5 to 2 liters	1
1 to 1.5 liters	0
0 to 1 liters	-1

Food Scoring Scale

Meal Quality	Score
Meal does not exist	1
Healthy and in reasonable quantity	2
Healthy but in excess	1
Neutral meal	0
Unhealthy meal	-1
Unhealthy and in excess	-2
Includes ice cream, cakes, soft drinks, or French fries	-1 per item

Physical Activity Scoring Scale

Activity Type	Score
Walking – 15 minutes	1
Running – 10 minutes	1
Other intense activities – 10 minutes	1
Sitting – every 2 hours continuously	-1

Daily Score

| Water Intake | + | Break fast | Morning snack | Lunch | Afternoon snack | Dinner | + | Physical Activity | = | ◯ |

Water Intake	Break fast	Morning snack	Lunch	Afternoon snack	Dinner	Physical Activity	
2	2	2	2	2	2	4	+13 to +16 Excellent
1	1	1	1	1	1	3	+9 to +12.9 Very Good
							+5 to +8.9 Good
0	0	0	0	0	0	2	+1 to +4.9 Neutral
							0 to -4.9 Poor
-1	-1	-1	-1	-1	-1	1	-5 to -8.9 Very Poor
							-9 to -15 Critical
	-2	-2	-2	-2	-2	0	
						-1	
						-2	
						-3	
						-4	

Hydration Scoring Scale

Water Intake (per day)*	Score
≥ 2.0 to 2.5 liters	2
1.5 to 2 liters	1
1 to 1.5 liters	0
0 to 1 liters	-1

Food Scoring Scale

Meal Quality	Score
Meal does not exist	1
Healthy and in reasonable quantity	2
Healthy but in excess	1
Neutral meal	0
Unhealthy meal	-1
Unhealthy and in excess	-2
Includes ice cream, cakes, soft drinks, or French fries	-1 per item

Physical Activity Scoring Scale

Activity Type	Score
Walking – 15 minutes	1
Running – 10 minutes	1
Other intense activities – 10 minutes	1
Sitting – every 2 hours continuously	-1

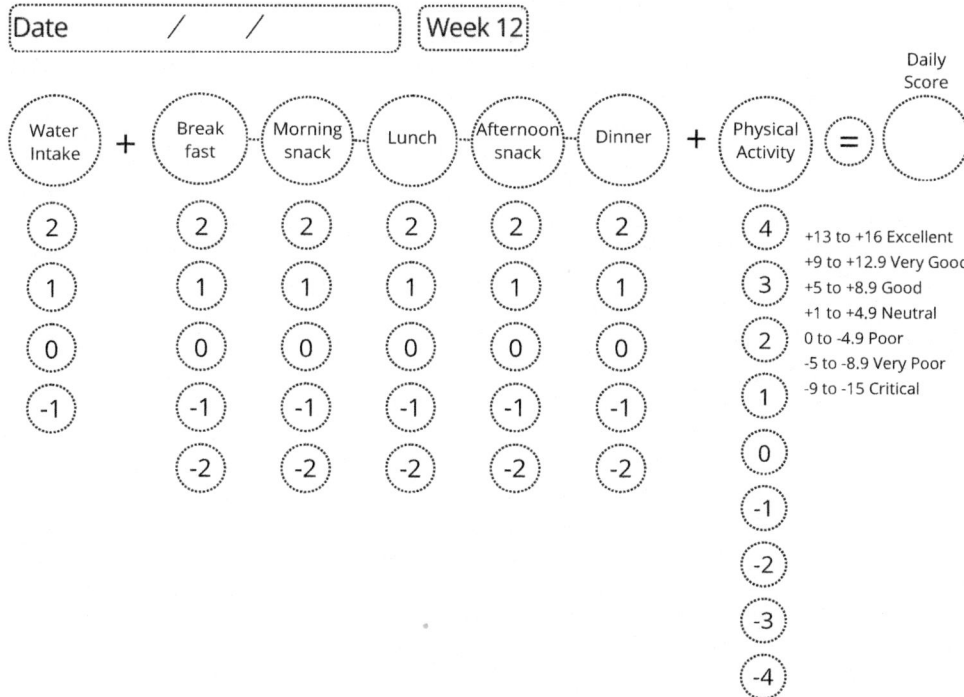

| Date | / | / | | Week 12 |

Water Intake + Break fast — Morning snack — Lunch — Afternoon snack — Dinner + Physical Activity = Daily Score

Water Intake: 2, 1, 0, -1

Break fast: 2, 1, 0, -1, -2

Morning snack: 2, 1, 0, -1, -2

Lunch: 2, 1, 0, -1, -2

Afternoon snack: 2, 1, 0, -1, -2

Dinner: 2, 1, 0, -1, -2

Physical Activity: 4, 3, 2, 1, 0, -1, -2, -3, -4

+13 to +16 Excellent
+9 to +12.9 Very Good
+5 to +8.9 Good
+1 to +4.9 Neutral
0 to -4.9 Poor
-5 to -8.9 Very Poor
-9 to -15 Critical

End of Week 12 – Weekly Summary

Twelve weeks of effort, discipline, and growth. Celebrate how far you've come — and keep going!

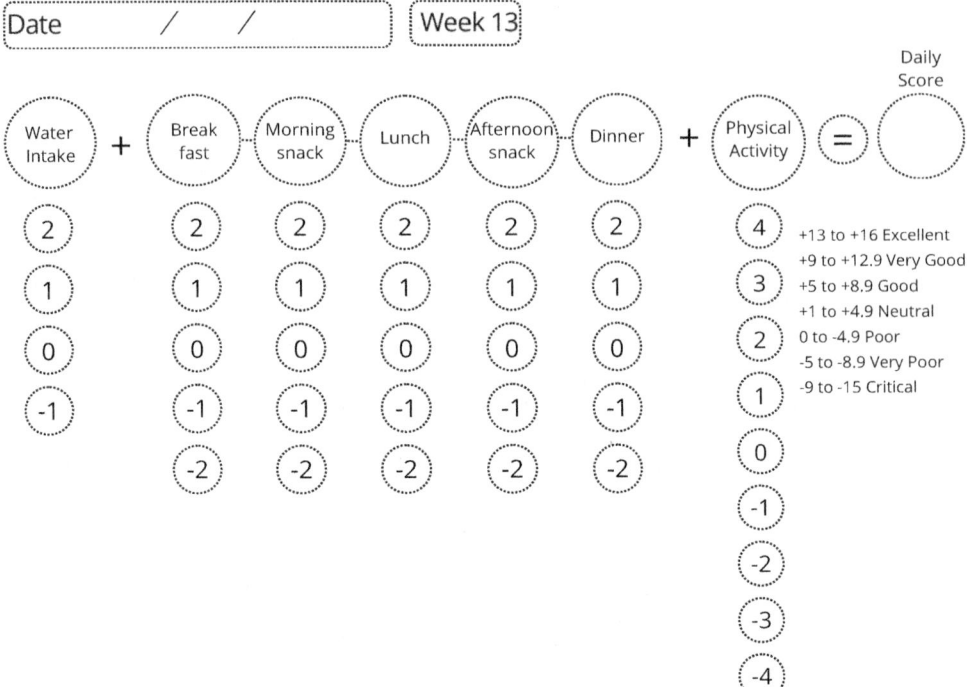

Water Intake + Breakfast · Morning snack · Lunch · Afternoon snack · Dinner + Physical Activity = Daily Score

+13 to +16 Excellent
+9 to +12.9 Very Good
+5 to +8.9 Good
+1 to +4.9 Neutral
0 to -4.9 Poor
-5 to -8.9 Very Poor
-9 to -15 Critical

Hydration Scoring Scale

Water Intake (per day)*	Score
≥ 2.0 to 2.5 liters	2
1.5 to 2 liters	1
1 to 1.5 liters	0
0 to 1 liters	-1

Food Scoring Scale

Meal Quality	Score
Meal does not exist	1
Healthy and in reasonable quantity	2
Healthy but in excess	1
Neutral meal	0
Unhealthy meal	-1
Unhealthy and in excess	-2
Includes ice cream, cakes, soft drinks, or French fries	-1 per item

Physical Activity Scoring Scale

Activity Type	Score
Walking – 15 minutes	1
Running – 10 minutes	1
Other intense activities – 10 minutes	1
Sitting – every 2 hours continuously	-1

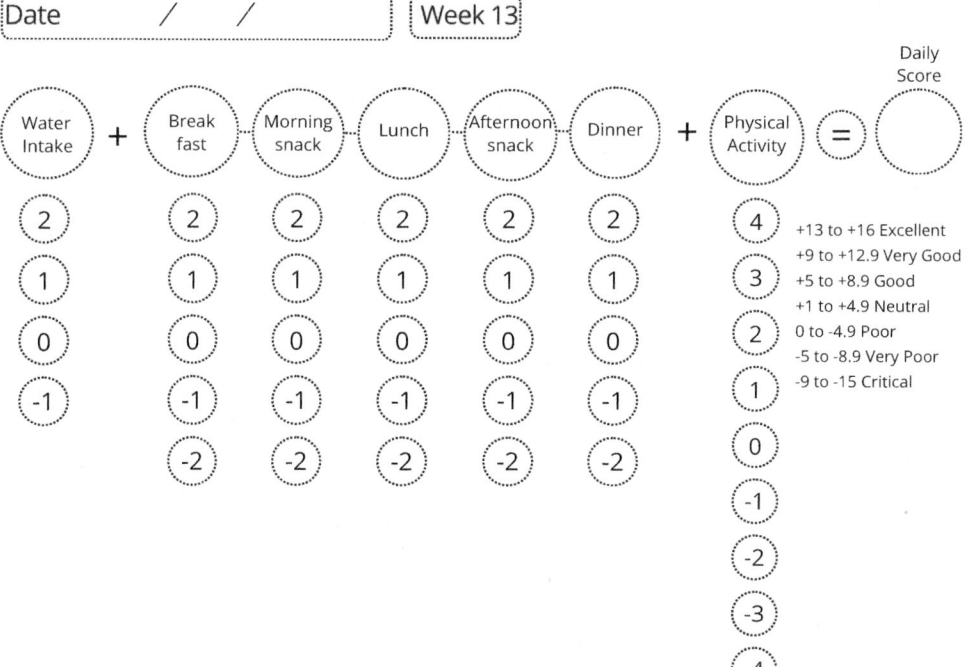

Date / /	Week 13

Water Intake + Break fast / Morning snack (Lunch / Afternoon snack / Dinner) + Physical Activity = Daily Score

Water Intake: 2, 1, 0, -1

Breakfast: 2, 1, 0, -1, -2

Morning snack: 2, 1, 0, -1, -2

Lunch: 2, 1, 0, -1, -2

Afternoon snack: 2, 1, 0, -1, -2

Dinner: 2, 1, 0, -1, -2

Physical Activity: 4, 3, 2, 1, 0, -1, -2, -3, -4

+13 to +16 Excellent
+9 to +12.9 Very Good
+5 to +8.9 Good
+1 to +4.9 Neutral
0 to -4.9 Poor
-5 to -8.9 Very Poor
-9 to -15 Critical

Hydration Scoring Scale

Water Intake (per day)*	Score
≥ 2.0 to 2.5 liters	2
1.5 to 2 liters	1
1 to 1.5 liters	0
0 to 1 liters	-1

Food Scoring Scale

Meal Quality	Score
Meal does not exist	1
Healthy and in reasonable quantity	2
Healthy but in excess	1
Neutral meal	0
Unhealthy meal	-1
Unhealthy and in excess	-2
Includes ice cream, cakes, soft drinks, or French fries	-1 per item

Physical Activity Scoring Scale

Activity Type	Score
Walking – 15 minutes	1
Running – 10 minutes	1
Other intense activities – 10 minutes	1
Sitting – every 2 hours continuously	-1

Daily Score

(Water Intake) + (Break fast) (Morning snack) (Lunch) (Afternoon snack) (Dinner) + (Physical Activity) (=) ( )

Water Intake	Break fast	Morning snack	Lunch	Afternoon snack	Dinner		Physical Activity
2	2	2	2	2	2		4
1	1	1	1	1	1		3
0	0	0	0	0	0		2
-1	-1	-1	-1	-1	-1		1
	-2	-2	-2	-2	-2		0
							-1
							-2
							-3
							-4

+13 to +16 Excellent
+9 to +12.9 Very Good
+5 to +8.9 Good
+1 to +4.9 Neutral
0 to -4.9 Poor
-5 to -8.9 Very Poor
-9 to -15 Critical

Hydration Scoring Scale

Water Intake (per day)*	Score
≥ 2.0 to 2.5 liters	2
1.5 to 2 liters	1
1 to 1.5 liters	0
0 to 1 liters	-1

Food Scoring Scale

Meal Quality	Score
Meal does not exist	1
Healthy and in reasonable quantity	2
Healthy but in excess	1
Neutral meal	0
Unhealthy meal	-1
Unhealthy and in excess	-2
Includes ice cream, cakes, soft drinks, or French fries	-1 per item

Physical Activity Scoring Scale

Activity Type	Score
Walking – 15 minutes	1
Running – 10 minutes	1
Other intense activities – 10 minutes	1
Sitting – every 2 hours continuously	-1

Date _____ / _____ / _____   Week 13

Water Intake + Break fast   Morning snack   Lunch   Afternoon snack   Dinner + Physical Activity = Daily Score

Water Intake	Breakfast	Morning snack	Lunch	Afternoon snack	Dinner	Physical Activity
2	2	2	2	2	2	4
1	1	1	1	1	1	3
0	0	0	0	0	0	2
-1	-1	-1	-1	-1	-1	1
	-2	-2	-2	-2	-2	0
						-1
						-2
						-3
						-4

+13 to +16 Excellent
+9 to +12.9 Very Good
+5 to +8.9 Good
+1 to +4.9 Neutral
0 to -4.9 Poor
-5 to -8.9 Very Poor
-9 to -15 Critical

Hydration Scoring Scale

Water Intake (per day)*	Score
≥ 2.0 to 2.5 liters	2
1.5 to 2 liters	1
1 to 1.5 liters	0
0 to 1 liters	-1

Food Scoring Scale

Meal Quality	Score
Meal does not exist	1
Healthy and in reasonable quantity	2
Healthy but in excess	1
Neutral meal	0
Unhealthy meal	-1
Unhealthy and in excess	-2
Includes ice cream, cakes, soft drinks, or French fries	-1 per item

Physical Activity Scoring Scale

Activity Type	Score
Walking – 15 minutes	1
Running – 10 minutes	1
Other intense activities – 10 minutes	1
Sitting – every 2 hours continuously	-1

Daily Score

(Water Intake) + (Break fast) (Morning snack) (Lunch) (Afternoon snack) (Dinner) + (Physical Activity) = ( )

Water Intake	Break fast	Morning snack	Lunch	Afternoon snack	Dinner	Physical Activity
2	2	2	2	2	2	4
1	1	1	1	1	1	3
0	0	0	0	0	0	2
-1	-1	-1	-1	-1	-1	1
	-2	-2	-2	-2	-2	0
						-1
						-2
						-3
						-4

+13 to +16 Excellent
+9 to +12.9 Very Good
+5 to +8.9 Good
+1 to +4.9 Neutral
0 to -4.9 Poor
-5 to -8.9 Very Poor
-9 to -15 Critical

Hydration Scoring Scale

Water Intake (per day)*	Score
≥ 2.0 to 2.5 liters	2
1.5 to 2 liters	1
1 to 1.5 liters	0
0 to 1 liters	-1

Food Scoring Scale

Meal Quality	Score
Meal does not exist	1
Healthy and in reasonable quantity	2
Healthy but in excess	1
Neutral meal	0
Unhealthy meal	-1
Unhealthy and in excess	-2
Includes ice cream, cakes, soft drinks, or French fries	-1 per item

Physical Activity Scoring Scale

Activity Type	Score
Walking – 15 minutes	1
Running – 10 minutes	1
Other intense activities – 10 minutes	1
Sitting – every 2 hours continuously	-1

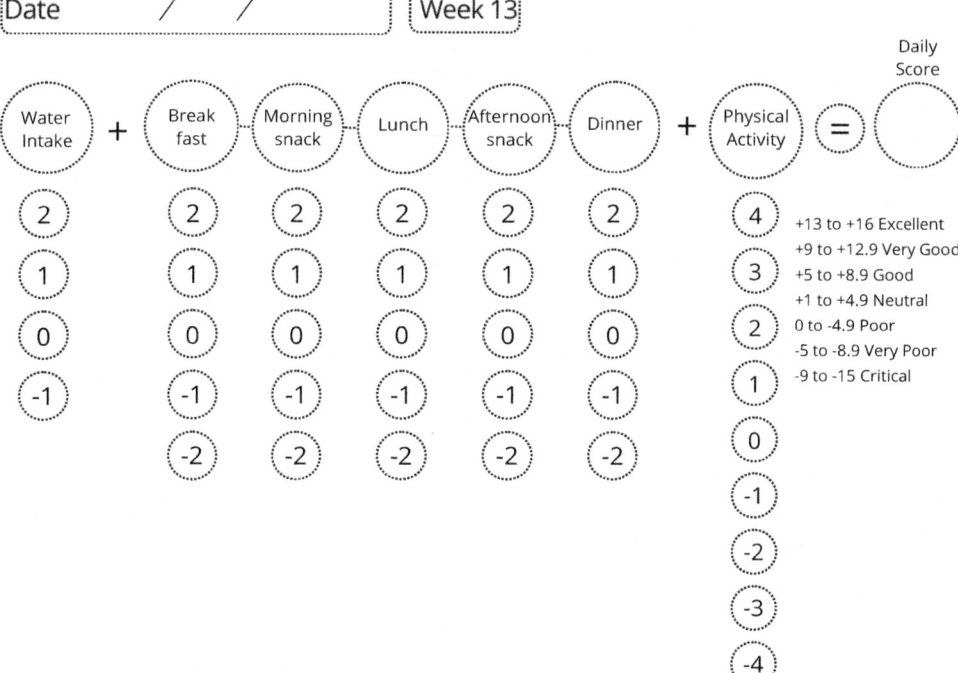

+13 to +16 Excellent
+9 to +12.9 Very Good
+5 to +8.9 Good
+1 to +4.9 Neutral
0 to -4.9 Poor
-5 to -8.9 Very Poor
-9 to -15 Critical

Hydration Scoring Scale

Water Intake (per day)*	Score
≥ 2.0 to 2.5 liters	2
1.5 to 2 liters	1
1 to 1.5 liters	0
0 to 1 liters	-1

Food Scoring Scale

Meal Quality	Score
Meal does not exist	1
Healthy and in reasonable quantity	2
Healthy but in excess	1
Neutral meal	0
Unhealthy meal	-1
Unhealthy and in excess	-2
Includes ice cream, cakes, soft drinks, or French fries	-1 per item

Physical Activity Scoring Scale

Activity Type	Score
Walking – 15 minutes	1
Running – 10 minutes	1
Other intense activities – 10 minutes	1
Sitting – every 2 hours continuously	-1

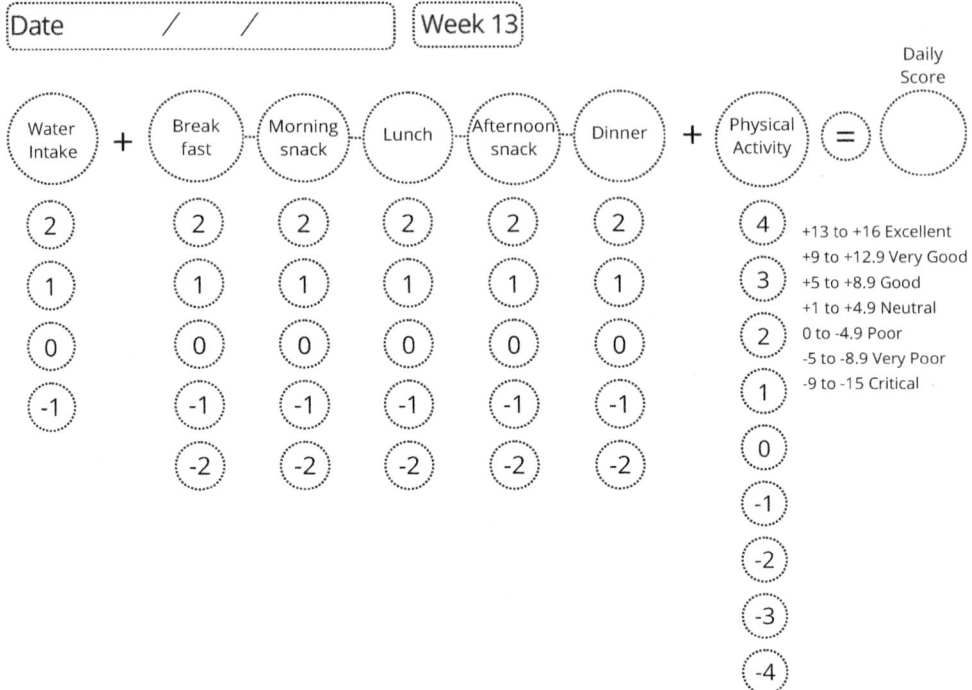

Date　　　/　　/　　Week 13

Water Intake + Break fast / Morning snack / Lunch / Afternoon snack / Dinner + Physical Activity = Daily Score

Water Intake: 2, 1, 0, -1

Breakfast: 2, 1, 0, -1, -2

Morning snack: 2, 1, 0, -1, -2

Lunch: 2, 1, 0, -1, -2

Afternoon snack: 2, 1, 0, -1, -2

Dinner: 2, 1, 0, -1, -2

Physical Activity: 4, 3, 2, 1, 0, -1, -2, -3, -4

+13 to +16 Excellent
+9 to +12.9 Very Good
+5 to +8.9 Good
+1 to +4.9 Neutral
0 to -4.9 Poor
-5 to -8.9 Very Poor
-9 to -15 Critical

End of Week 13 – Weekly Summary

This isn't just a habit anymore — it's who you're becoming. Keep choosing the person you want to be.

Daily Score

(Water Intake) + (Break fast) (Morning snack) (Lunch) (Afternoon snack) (Dinner) + (Physical Activity) = ( )

Water Intake	Break fast	Morning snack	Lunch	Afternoon snack	Dinner	Physical Activity
2	2	2	2	2	2	4
1	1	1	1	1	1	3
0	0	0	0	0	0	2
-1	-1	-1	-1	-1	-1	1
	-2	-2	-2	-2	-2	0
						-1
						-2
						-3
						-4

+13 to +16 Excellent
+9 to +12.9 Very Good
+5 to +8.9 Good
+1 to +4.9 Neutral
0 to -4.9 Poor
-5 to -8.9 Very Poor
-9 to -15 Critical

Hydration Scoring Scale

Water Intake (per day)*	Score
≥ 2.0 to 2.5 liters	2
1.5 to 2 liters	1
1 to 1.5 liters	0
0 to 1 liters	-1

Food Scoring Scale

Meal Quality	Score
Meal does not exist	1
Healthy and in reasonable quantity	2
Healthy but in excess	1
Neutral meal	0
Unhealthy meal	-1
Unhealthy and in excess	-2
Includes ice cream, cakes, soft drinks, or French fries	-1 per item

Physical Activity Scoring Scale

Activity Type	Score
Walking – 15 minutes	1
Running – 10 minutes	1
Other intense activities – 10 minutes	1
Sitting – every 2 hours continuously	-1

Daily Score

Water Intake + Break fast — Morning snack — Lunch — Afternoon snack — Dinner + Physical Activity = ( )

Water Intake	Break fast	Morning snack	Lunch	Afternoon snack	Dinner	Physical Activity
2	2	2	2	2	2	4
1	1	1	1	1	1	3
0	0	0	0	0	0	2
-1	-1	-1	-1	-1	-1	1
	-2	-2	-2	-2	-2	0
						-1
						-2
						-3
						-4

+13 to +16 Excellent
+9 to +12.9 Very Good
+5 to +8.9 Good
+1 to +4.9 Neutral
0 to -4.9 Poor
-5 to -8.9 Very Poor
-9 to -15 Critical

Hydration Scoring Scale

Water Intake (per day)*	Score
≥ 2.0 to 2.5 liters	2
1.5 to 2 liters	1
1 to 1.5 liters	0
0 to 1 liters	-1

Food Scoring Scale

Meal Quality	Score
Meal does not exist	1
Healthy and in reasonable quantity	2
Healthy but in excess	1
Neutral meal	0
Unhealthy meal	-1
Unhealthy and in excess	-2
Includes ice cream, cakes, soft drinks, or French fries	-1 per item

Physical Activity Scoring Scale

Activity Type	Score
Walking – 15 minutes	1
Running – 10 minutes	1
Other intense activities – 10 minutes	1
Sitting – every 2 hours continuously	-1

Daily Score

(Water Intake) + (Break fast) (Morning snack) (Lunch) (Afternoon snack) (Dinner) + (Physical Activity) = ( )

Water Intake: 2, 1, 0, -1

Breakfast: 2, 1, 0, -1, -2

Morning snack: 2, 1, 0, -1, -2

Lunch: 2, 1, 0, -1, -2

Afternoon snack: 2, 1, 0, -1, -2

Dinner: 2, 1, 0, -1, -2

Physical Activity: 4, 3, 2, 1, 0, -1, -2, -3, -4

+13 to +16 Excellent
+9 to +12.9 Very Good
+5 to +8.9 Good
+1 to +4.9 Neutral
0 to -4.9 Poor
-5 to -8.9 Very Poor
-9 to -15 Critical

Hydration Scoring Scale

Water Intake (per day)*	Score
≥ 2.0 to 2.5 liters	2
1.5 to 2 liters	1
1 to 1.5 liters	0
0 to 1 liters	-1

Food Scoring Scale

Meal Quality	Score
Meal does not exist	1
Healthy and in reasonable quantity	2
Healthy but in excess	1
Neutral meal	0
Unhealthy meal	-1
Unhealthy and in excess	-2
Includes ice cream, cakes, soft drinks, or French fries	-1 per item

Physical Activity Scoring Scale

Activity Type	Score
Walking – 15 minutes	1
Running – 10 minutes	1
Other intense activities – 10 minutes	1
Sitting – every 2 hours continuously	-1

Daily Score

Water Intake + Break fast · Morning snack · Lunch · Afternoon snack · Dinner + Physical Activity = ( )

Water Intake: 2, 1, 0, -1

Break fast: 2, 1, 0, -1, -2

Morning snack: 2, 1, 0, -1, -2

Lunch: 2, 1, 0, -1, -2

Afternoon snack: 2, 1, 0, -1, -2

Dinner: 2, 1, 0, -1, -2

Physical Activity: 4, 3, 2, 1, 0, -1, -2, -3, -4

+13 to +16 Excellent
+9 to +12.9 Very Good
+5 to +8.9 Good
+1 to +4.9 Neutral
0 to -4.9 Poor
-5 to -8.9 Very Poor
-9 to -15 Critical

Hydration Scoring Scale

Water Intake (per day)*	Score
≥ 2.0 to 2.5 liters	2
1.5 to 2 liters	1
1 to 1.5 liters	0
0 to 1 liters	-1

Food Scoring Scale

Meal Quality	Score
Meal does not exist	1
Healthy and in reasonable quantity	2
Healthy but in excess	1
Neutral meal	0
Unhealthy meal	-1
Unhealthy and in excess	-2
Includes ice cream, cakes, soft drinks, or French fries	-1 per item

Physical Activity Scoring Scale

Activity Type	Score
Walking – 15 minutes	1
Running – 10 minutes	1
Other intense activities – 10 minutes	1
Sitting – every 2 hours continuously	-1

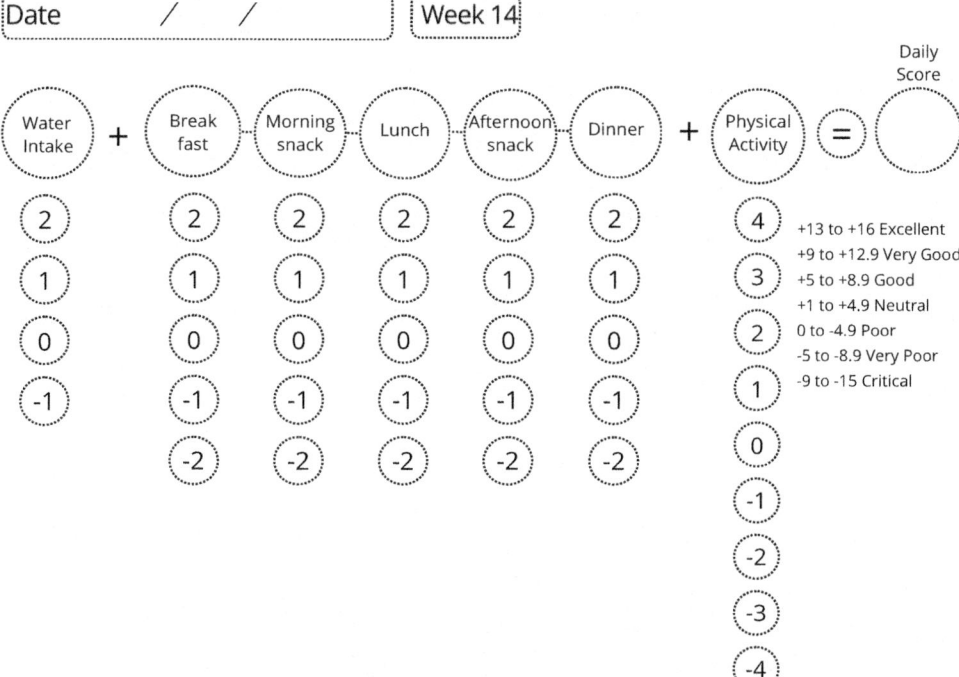

Water Intake + Break fast + Morning snack + Lunch + Afternoon snack + Dinner + Physical Activity = Daily Score

+13 to +16 Excellent
+9 to +12.9 Very Good
+5 to +8.9 Good
+1 to +4.9 Neutral
0 to -4.9 Poor
-5 to -8.9 Very Poor
-9 to -15 Critical

Hydration Scoring Scale

Water Intake (per day)*	Score
≥ 2.0 to 2.5 liters	2
1.5 to 2 liters	1
1 to 1.5 liters	0
0 to 1 liters	-1

Food Scoring Scale

Meal Quality	Score
Meal does not exist	1
Healthy and in reasonable quantity	2
Healthy but in excess	1
Neutral meal	0
Unhealthy meal	-1
Unhealthy and in excess	-2
Includes ice cream, cakes, soft drinks, or French fries	-1 per item

Physical Activity Scoring Scale

Activity Type	Score
Walking – 15 minutes	1
Running – 10 minutes	1
Other intense activities – 10 minutes	1
Sitting – every 2 hours continuously	-1

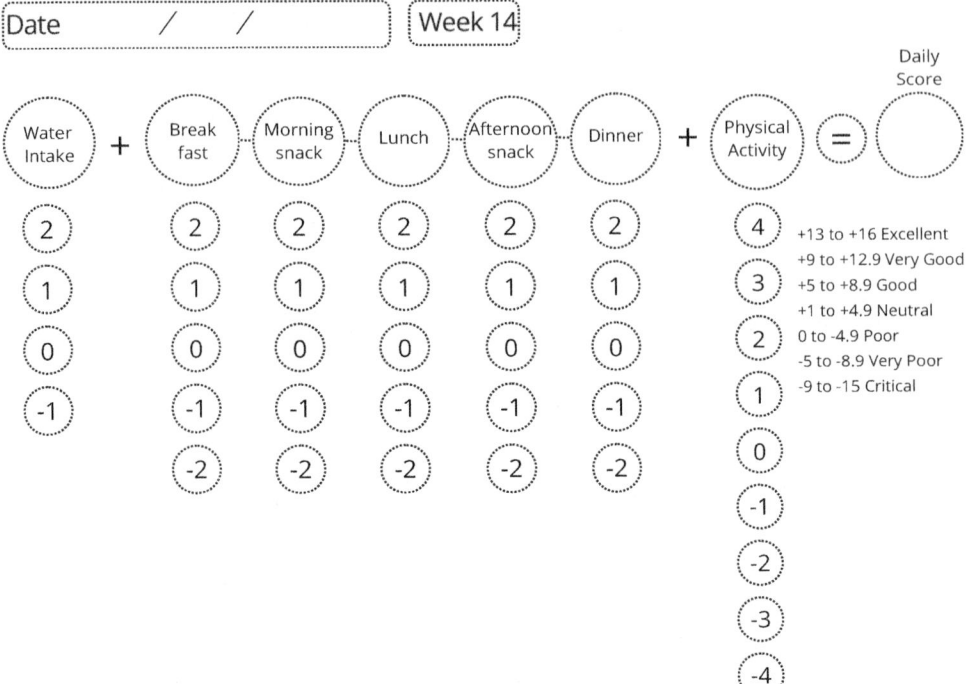

Date _____ / _____ / _____   Week 14

Water Intake + Breakfast Morning snack Lunch Afternoon snack Dinner + Physical Activity = Daily Score

Water Intake: 2, 1, 0, -1

Breakfast: 2, 1, 0, -1, -2

Morning snack: 2, 1, 0, -1, -2

Lunch: 2, 1, 0, -1, -2

Afternoon snack: 2, 1, 0, -1, -2

Dinner: 2, 1, 0, -1, -2

Physical Activity: 4, 3, 2, 1, 0, -1, -2, -3, -4

+13 to +16 Excellent
+9 to +12.9 Very Good
+5 to +8.9 Good
+1 to +4.9 Neutral
0 to -4.9 Poor
-5 to -8.9 Very Poor
-9 to -15 Critical

Hydration Scoring Scale

Water Intake (per day)*	Score
≥ 2.0 to 2.5 liters	2
1.5 to 2 liters	1
1 to 1.5 liters	0
0 to 1 liters	-1

Food Scoring Scale

Meal Quality	Score
Meal does not exist	1
Healthy and in reasonable quantity	2
Healthy but in excess	1
Neutral meal	0
Unhealthy meal	-1
Unhealthy and in excess	-2
Includes ice cream, cakes, soft drinks, or French fries	-1 per item

Physical Activity Scoring Scale

Activity Type	Score
Walking – 15 minutes	1
Running – 10 minutes	1
Other intense activities – 10 minutes	1
Sitting – every 2 hours continuously	-1

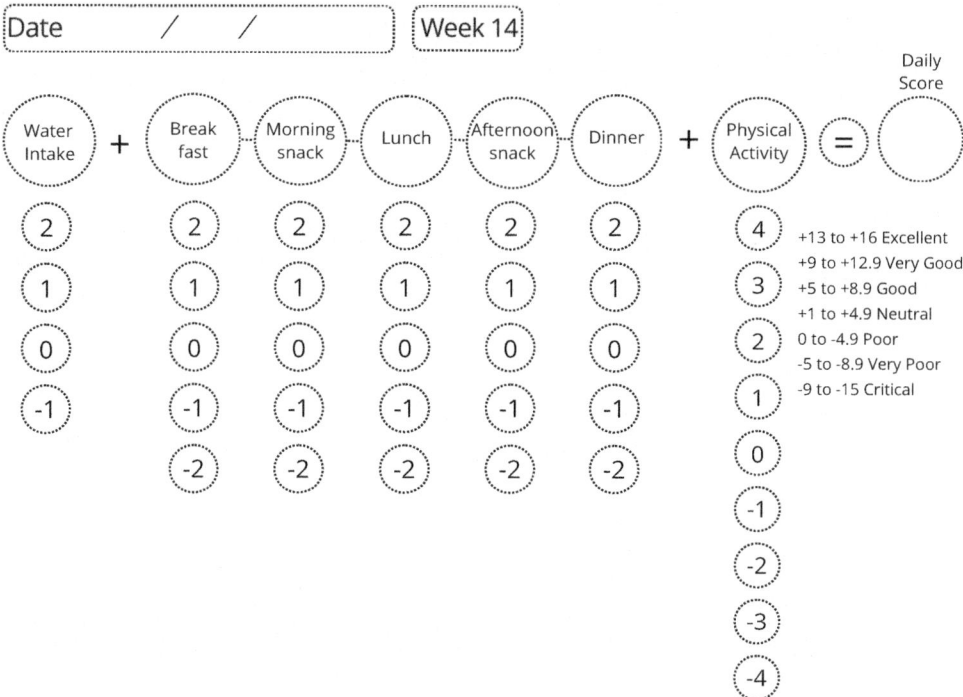

Date ___ / ___ / ___   Week 14

Daily Score

Water Intake + Breakfast / Morning snack / Lunch / Afternoon snack / Dinner + Physical Activity = ( )

Water Intake	Breakfast	Morning snack	Lunch	Afternoon snack	Dinner	Physical Activity
2	2	2	2	2	2	4
1	1	1	1	1	1	3
0	0	0	0	0	0	2
-1	-1	-1	-1	-1	-1	1
	-2	-2	-2	-2	-2	0

+13 to +16 Excellent
+9 to +12.9 Very Good
+5 to +8.9 Good
+1 to +4.9 Neutral
0 to -4.9 Poor
-5 to -8.9 Very Poor
-9 to -15 Critical

Physical Activity: -1, -2, -3, -4

End of Week 14 – Weekly Summary

Small wins stacked consistently create big results. Keep stacking — your journey is paying off.

Daily Score

Water Intake + Break fast — Morning snack — Lunch — Afternoon snack — Dinner + Physical Activity =

Water Intake	Break fast	Morning snack	Lunch	Afternoon snack	Dinner	Physical Activity
2	2	2	2	2	2	4
1	1	1	1	1	1	3
0	0	0	0	0	0	2
-1	-1	-1	-1	-1	-1	1
	-2	-2	-2	-2	-2	0
						-1
						-2
						-3
						-4

+13 to +16 Excellent
+9 to +12.9 Very Good
+5 to +8.9 Good
+1 to +4.9 Neutral
0 to -4.9 Poor
-5 to -8.9 Very Poor
-9 to -15 Critical

Hydration Scoring Scale

Water Intake (per day)*	Score
≥ 2.0 to 2.5 liters	2
1.5 to 2 liters	1
1 to 1.5 liters	0
0 to 1 liters	-1

Food Scoring Scale

Meal Quality	Score
Meal does not exist	1
Healthy and in reasonable quantity	2
Healthy but in excess	1
Neutral meal	0
Unhealthy meal	-1
Unhealthy and in excess	-2
Includes ice cream, cakes, soft drinks, or French fries	-1 per item

Physical Activity Scoring Scale

Activity Type	Score
Walking – 15 minutes	1
Running – 10 minutes	1
Other intense activities – 10 minutes	1
Sitting – every 2 hours continuously	-1

Daily
Score

Water Intake + Break fast · Morning snack · Lunch · Afternoon snack · Dinner + Physical Activity = ( )

Water Intake	Break fast	Morning snack	Lunch	Afternoon snack	Dinner	Physical Activity
2	2	2	2	2	2	4
1	1	1	1	1	1	3
0	0	0	0	0	0	2
-1	-1	-1	-1	-1	-1	1
	-2	-2	-2	-2	-2	0
						-1
						-2
						-3
						-4

+13 to +16 Excellent
+9 to +12.9 Very Good
+5 to +8.9 Good
+1 to +4.9 Neutral
0 to -4.9 Poor
-5 to -8.9 Very Poor
-9 to -15 Critical

Hydration Scoring Scale

Water Intake (per day)*	Score
≥ 2.0 to 2.5 liters	2
1.5 to 2 liters	1
1 to 1.5 liters	0
0 to 1 liters	-1

Food Scoring Scale

Meal Quality	Score
Meal does not exist	1
Healthy and in reasonable quantity	2
Healthy but in excess	1
Neutral meal	0
Unhealthy meal	-1
Unhealthy and in excess	-2
Includes ice cream, cakes, soft drinks, or French fries	-1 per item

Physical Activity Scoring Scale

Activity Type	Score
Walking – 15 minutes	1
Running – 10 minutes	1
Other intense activities – 10 minutes	1
Sitting – every 2 hours continuously	-1

Water Intake	+	Break fast	Morning snack	Lunch	Afternoon snack	Dinner	+	Physical Activity	=	Daily Score

Water Intake	Break fast	Morning snack	Lunch	Afternoon snack	Dinner	Physical Activity	
2	2	2	2	2	2	4	+13 to +16 Excellent
1	1	1	1	1	1	3	+9 to +12.9 Very Good
0	0	0	0	0	0	2	+5 to +8.9 Good
-1	-1	-1	-1	-1	-1	1	+1 to +4.9 Neutral
	-2	-2	-2	-2	-2	0	0 to -4.9 Poor
						-1	-5 to -8.9 Very Poor
						-2	-9 to -15 Critical
						-3	
						-4	

Hydration Scoring Scale

Water Intake (per day)*	Score
≥ 2.0 to 2.5 liters	2
1.5 to 2 liters	1
1 to 1.5 liters	0
0 to 1 liters	-1

Food Scoring Scale

Meal Quality	Score
Meal does not exist	1
Healthy and in reasonable quantity	2
Healthy but in excess	1
Neutral meal	0
Unhealthy meal	-1
Unhealthy and in excess	-2
Includes ice cream, cakes, soft drinks, or French fries	-1 per item

Physical Activity Scoring Scale

Activity Type	Score
Walking – 15 minutes	1
Running – 10 minutes	1
Other intense activities – 10 minutes	1
Sitting – every 2 hours continuously	-1

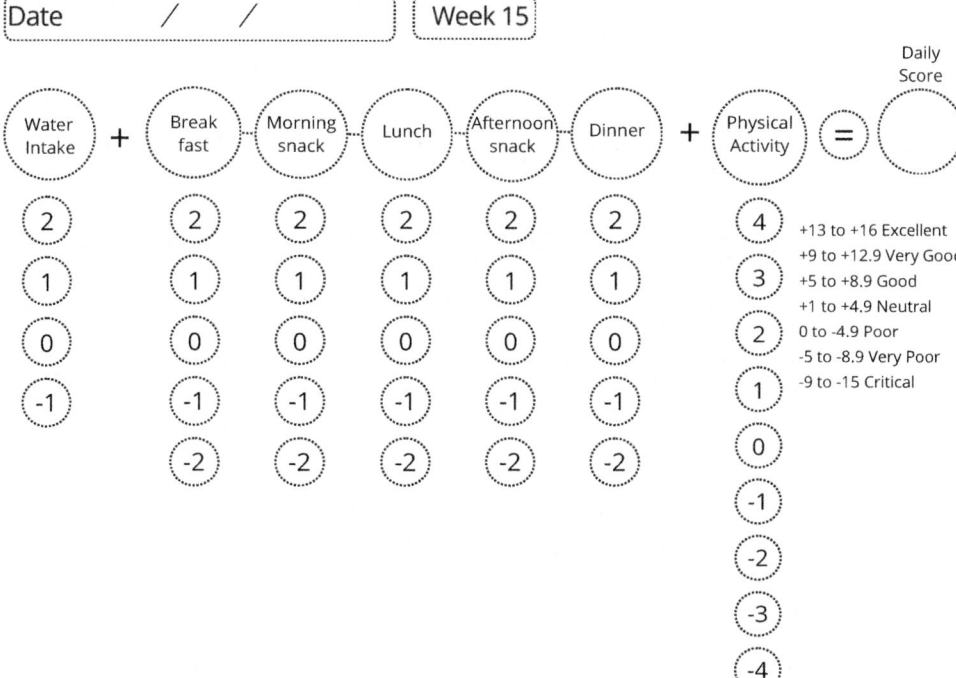

Daily Score

Water Intake + Break fast | Morning snack | Lunch | Afternoon snack | Dinner + Physical Activity = ( )

+13 to +16 Excellent
+9 to +12.9 Very Good
+5 to +8.9 Good
+1 to +4.9 Neutral
0 to -4.9 Poor
-5 to -8.9 Very Poor
-9 to -15 Critical

Hydration Scoring Scale

Water Intake (per day)*	Score
≥ 2.0 to 2.5 liters	2
1.5 to 2 liters	1
1 to 1.5 liters	0
0 to 1 liters	-1

Food Scoring Scale

Meal Quality	Score
Meal does not exist	1
Healthy and in reasonable quantity	2
Healthy but in excess	1
Neutral meal	0
Unhealthy meal	-1
Unhealthy and in excess	-2
Includes ice cream, cakes, soft drinks, or French fries	-1 per item

Physical Activity Scoring Scale

Activity Type	Score
Walking – 15 minutes	1
Running – 10 minutes	1
Other intense activities – 10 minutes	1
Sitting – every 2 hours continuously	-1

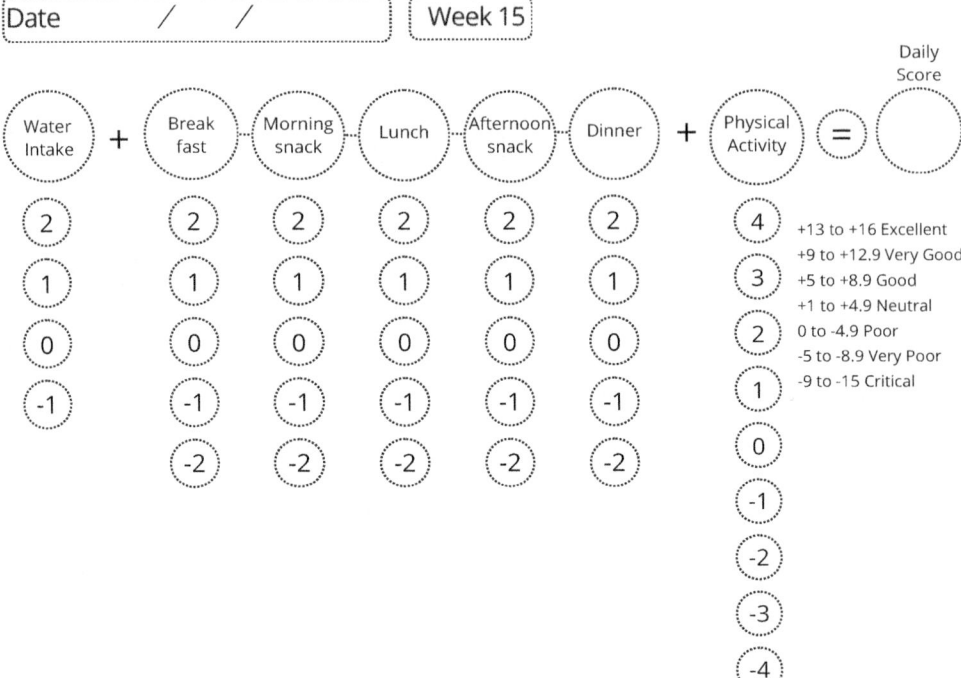

Daily Score

+13 to +16 Excellent
+9 to +12.9 Very Good
+5 to +8.9 Good
+1 to +4.9 Neutral
0 to -4.9 Poor
-5 to -8.9 Very Poor
-9 to -15 Critical

Hydration Scoring Scale

Water Intake (per day)*	Score
≥ 2.0 to 2.5 liters	2
1.5 to 2 liters	1
1 to 1.5 liters	0
0 to 1 liters	-1

Food Scoring Scale

Meal Quality	Score
Meal does not exist	1
Healthy and in reasonable quantity	2
Healthy but in excess	1
Neutral meal	0
Unhealthy meal	-1
Unhealthy and in excess	-2
Includes ice cream, cakes, soft drinks, or French fries	-1 per item

Physical Activity Scoring Scale

Activity Type	Score
Walking – 15 minutes	1
Running – 10 minutes	1
Other intense activities – 10 minutes	1
Sitting – every 2 hours continuously	-1

Water Intake + Breakfast · Morning snack · Lunch · Afternoon snack · Dinner + Physical Activity = Daily Score

Water Intake	Breakfast	Morning snack	Lunch	Afternoon snack	Dinner	Physical Activity
2	2	2	2	2	2	4
1	1	1	1	1	1	3
0	0	0	0	0	0	2
-1	-1	-1	-1	-1	-1	1
	-2	-2	-2	-2	-2	0
						-1
						-2
						-3
						-4

+13 to +16 Excellent
+9 to +12.9 Very Good
+5 to +8.9 Good
+1 to +4.9 Neutral
0 to -4.9 Poor
-5 to -8.9 Very Poor
-9 to -15 Critical

Hydration Scoring Scale

Water Intake (per day)*	Score
≥ 2.0 to 2.5 liters	2
1.5 to 2 liters	1
1 to 1.5 liters	0
0 to 1 liters	-1

Food Scoring Scale

Meal Quality	Score
Meal does not exist	1
Healthy and in reasonable quantity	2
Healthy but in excess	1
Neutral meal	0
Unhealthy meal	-1
Unhealthy and in excess	-2
Includes ice cream, cakes, soft drinks, or French fries	-1 per item

Physical Activity Scoring Scale

Activity Type	Score
Walking – 15 minutes	1
Running – 10 minutes	1
Other intense activities – 10 minutes	1
Sitting – every 2 hours continuously	-1

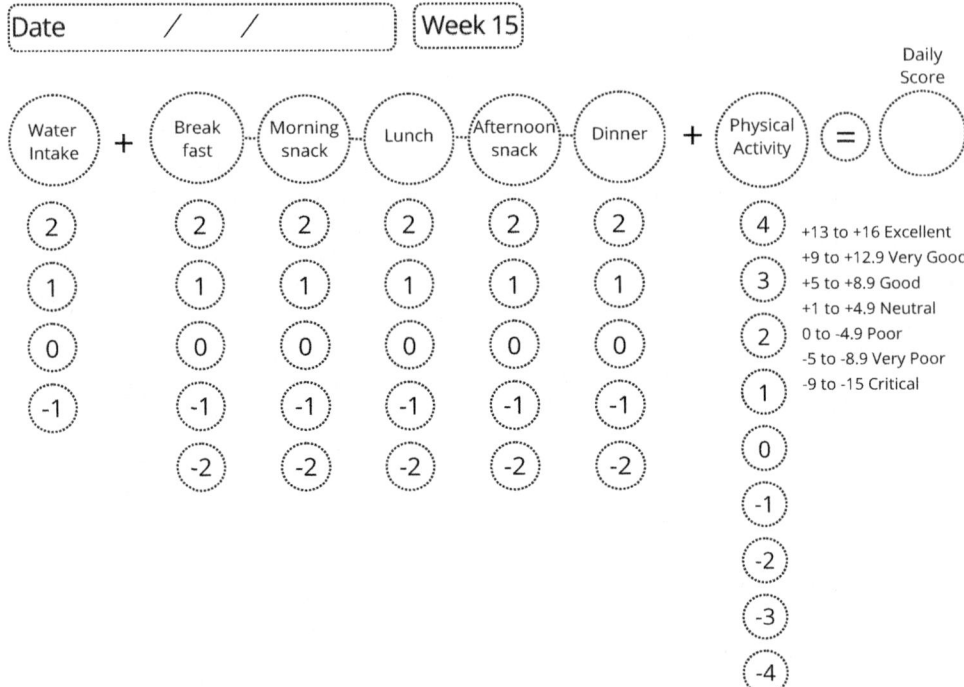

Date   /   /

Week 15

Daily Score

Water Intake + Break fast   Morning snack   Lunch   Afternoon snack   Dinner + Physical Activity = ◯

+13 to +16 Excellent
+9 to +12.9 Very Good
+5 to +8.9 Good
+1 to +4.9 Neutral
0 to -4.9 Poor
-5 to -8.9 Very Poor
-9 to -15 Critical

End of Week 15 – Weekly Summary

You're entering the final stretch. Stay focused, stay steady — lasting change is built in moments like these.

Daily Score

Water Intake + Break fast + Morning snack + Lunch + Afternoon snack + Dinner + Physical Activity =

Water Intake	Break fast	Morning snack	Lunch	Afternoon snack	Dinner	Physical Activity
2	2	2	2	2	2	4
1	1	1	1	1	1	3
0	0	0	0	0	0	2
-1	-1	-1	-1	-1	-1	1
	-2	-2	-2	-2	-2	0
						-1
						-2
						-3
						-4

+13 to +16 Excellent
+9 to +12.9 Very Good
+5 to +8.9 Good
+1 to +4.9 Neutral
0 to -4.9 Poor
-5 to -8.9 Very Poor
-9 to -15 Critical

Hydration Scoring Scale

Water Intake (per day)*	Score
≥ 2.0 to 2.5 liters	2
1.5 to 2 liters	1
1 to 1.5 liters	0
0 to 1 liters	-1

Food Scoring Scale

Meal Quality	Score
Meal does not exist	1
Healthy and in reasonable quantity	2
Healthy but in excess	1
Neutral meal	0
Unhealthy meal	-1
Unhealthy and in excess	-2
Includes ice cream, cakes, soft drinks, or French fries	-1 per item

Physical Activity Scoring Scale

Activity Type	Score
Walking – 15 minutes	1
Running – 10 minutes	1
Other intense activities – 10 minutes	1
Sitting – every 2 hours continuously	-1

Daily Score

(Water Intake) + (Break fast) (Morning snack) (Lunch) (Afternoon snack) (Dinner) + (Physical Activity) (=) ( )

Water Intake	Break fast	Morning snack	Lunch	Afternoon snack	Dinner	Physical Activity
2	2	2	2	2	2	4
1	1	1	1	1	1	3
0	0	0	0	0	0	2
-1	-1	-1	-1	-1	-1	1
	-2	-2	-2	-2	-2	0
						-1
						-2
						-3
						-4

+13 to +16 Excellent
+9 to +12.9 Very Good
+5 to +8.9 Good
+1 to +4.9 Neutral
0 to -4.9 Poor
-5 to -8.9 Very Poor
-9 to -15 Critical

Hydration Scoring Scale

Water Intake (per day)*	Score
≥ 2.0 to 2.5 liters	2
1.5 to 2 liters	1
1 to 1.5 liters	0
0 to 1 liters	-1

Food Scoring Scale

Meal Quality	Score
Meal does not exist	1
Healthy and in reasonable quantity	2
Healthy but in excess	1
Neutral meal	0
Unhealthy meal	-1
Unhealthy and in excess	-2
Includes ice cream, cakes, soft drinks, or French fries	-1 per item

Physical Activity Scoring Scale

Activity Type	Score
Walking – 15 minutes	1
Running – 10 minutes	1
Other intense activities – 10 minutes	1
Sitting – every 2 hours continuously	-1

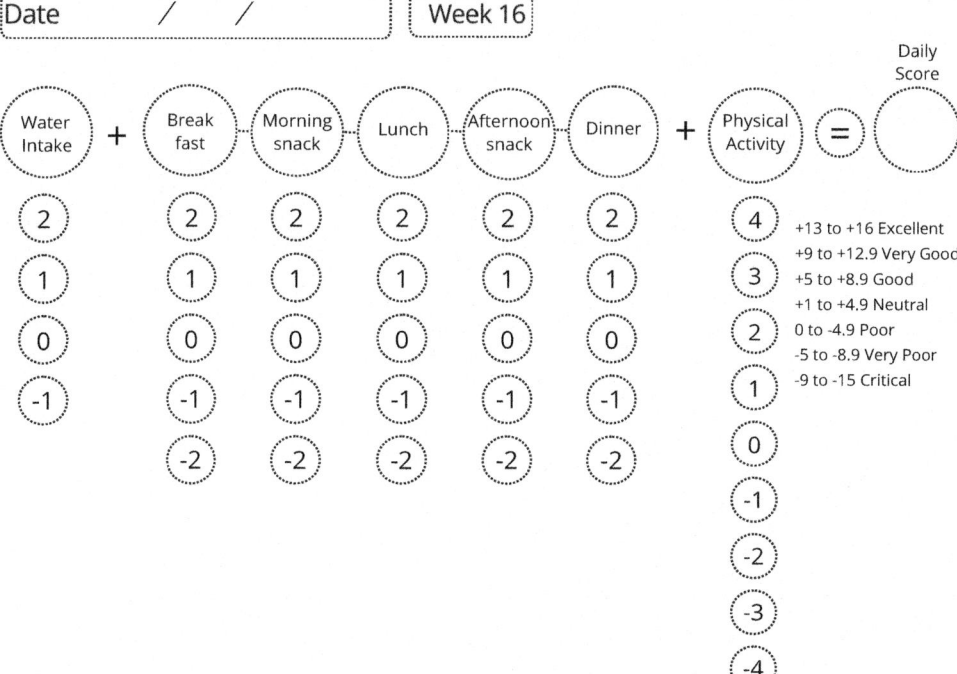

Hydration Scoring Scale	
Water Intake (per day)*	**Score**
≥ 2.0 to 2.5 liters	2
1.5 to 2 liters	1
1 to 1.5 liters	0
0 to 1 liters	-1

Food Scoring Scale	
Meal Quality	**Score**
Meal does not exist	1
Healthy and in reasonable quantity	2
Healthy but in excess	1
Neutral meal	0
Unhealthy meal	-1
Unhealthy and in excess	-2
Includes ice cream, cakes, soft drinks, or French fries	-1 per item

Physical Activity Scoring Scale	
Activity Type	**Score**
Walking – 15 minutes	1
Running – 10 minutes	1
Other intense activities – 10 minutes	1
Sitting – every 2 hours continuously	-1

Daily Score

Water Intake **+** Break fast — Morning snack — Lunch — Afternoon snack — Dinner **+** Physical Activity **=** ◯

Water Intake	Break fast	Morning snack	Lunch	Afternoon snack	Dinner	Physical Activity
2	2	2	2	2	2	4
1	1	1	1	1	1	3
0	0	0	0	0	0	2
-1	-1	-1	-1	-1	-1	1
	-2	-2	-2	-2	-2	0
						-1
						-2
						-3
						-4

+13 to +16 Excellent
+9 to +12.9 Very Good
+5 to +8.9 Good
+1 to +4.9 Neutral
0 to -4.9 Poor
-5 to -8.9 Very Poor
-9 to -15 Critical

Hydration Scoring Scale

Water Intake (per day)*	Score
≥ 2.0 to 2.5 liters	2
1.5 to 2 liters	1
1 to 1.5 liters	0
0 to 1 liters	-1

Food Scoring Scale

Meal Quality	Score
Meal does not exist	1
Healthy and in reasonable quantity	2
Healthy but in excess	1
Neutral meal	0
Unhealthy meal	-1
Unhealthy and in excess	-2
Includes ice cream, cakes, soft drinks, or French fries	-1 per item

Physical Activity Scoring Scale

Activity Type	Score
Walking – 15 minutes	1
Running – 10 minutes	1
Other intense activities – 10 minutes	1
Sitting – every 2 hours continuously	-1

Date	/	/		Week 16

Daily Score

Water Intake	+	Break fast	Morning snack	Lunch	Afternoon snack	Dinner	+	Physical Activity	=	

Water Intake: 2, 1, 0, -1

Break fast: 2, 1, 0, -1, -2

Morning snack: 2, 1, 0, -1, -2

Lunch: 2, 1, 0, -1, -2

Afternoon snack: 2, 1, 0, -1, -2

Dinner: 2, 1, 0, -1, -2

Physical Activity: 4, 3, 2, 1, 0, -1, -2, -3, -4

+13 to +16 Excellent
+9 to +12.9 Very Good
+5 to +8.9 Good
+1 to +4.9 Neutral
0 to -4.9 Poor
-5 to -8.9 Very Poor
-9 to -15 Critical

Hydration Scoring Scale

Water Intake (per day)*	Score
≥ 2.0 to 2.5 liters	2
1.5 to 2 liters	1
1 to 1.5 liters	0
0 to 1 liters	-1

Food Scoring Scale

Meal Quality	Score
Meal does not exist	1
Healthy and in reasonable quantity	2
Healthy but in excess	1
Neutral meal	0
Unhealthy meal	-1
Unhealthy and in excess	-2
Includes ice cream, cakes, soft drinks, or French fries	-1 per item

Physical Activity Scoring Scale

Activity Type	Score
Walking – 15 minutes	1
Running – 10 minutes	1
Other intense activities – 10 minutes	1
Sitting – every 2 hours continuously	-1

Daily Score

Water Intake + Break fast — Morning snack — Lunch — Afternoon snack — Dinner + Physical Activity = ( )

Water Intake	Break fast	Morning snack	Lunch	Afternoon snack	Dinner	Physical Activity
2	2	2	2	2	2	4
1	1	1	1	1	1	3
0	0	0	0	0	0	2
-1	-1	-1	-1	-1	-1	1
	-2	-2	-2	-2	-2	0
						-1
						-2
						-3
						-4

+13 to +16 Excellent
+9 to +12.9 Very Good
+5 to +8.9 Good
+1 to +4.9 Neutral
0 to -4.9 Poor
-5 to -8.9 Very Poor
-9 to -15 Critical

Hydration Scoring Scale

Water Intake (per day)*	Score
≥ 2.0 to 2.5 liters	2
1.5 to 2 liters	1
1 to 1.5 liters	0
0 to 1 liters	-1

Food Scoring Scale

Meal Quality	Score
Meal does not exist	1
Healthy and in reasonable quantity	2
Healthy but in excess	1
Neutral meal	0
Unhealthy meal	-1
Unhealthy and in excess	-2
Includes ice cream, cakes, soft drinks, or French fries	-1 per item

Physical Activity Scoring Scale

Activity Type	Score
Walking – 15 minutes	1
Running – 10 minutes	1
Other intense activities – 10 minutes	1
Sitting – every 2 hours continuously	-1

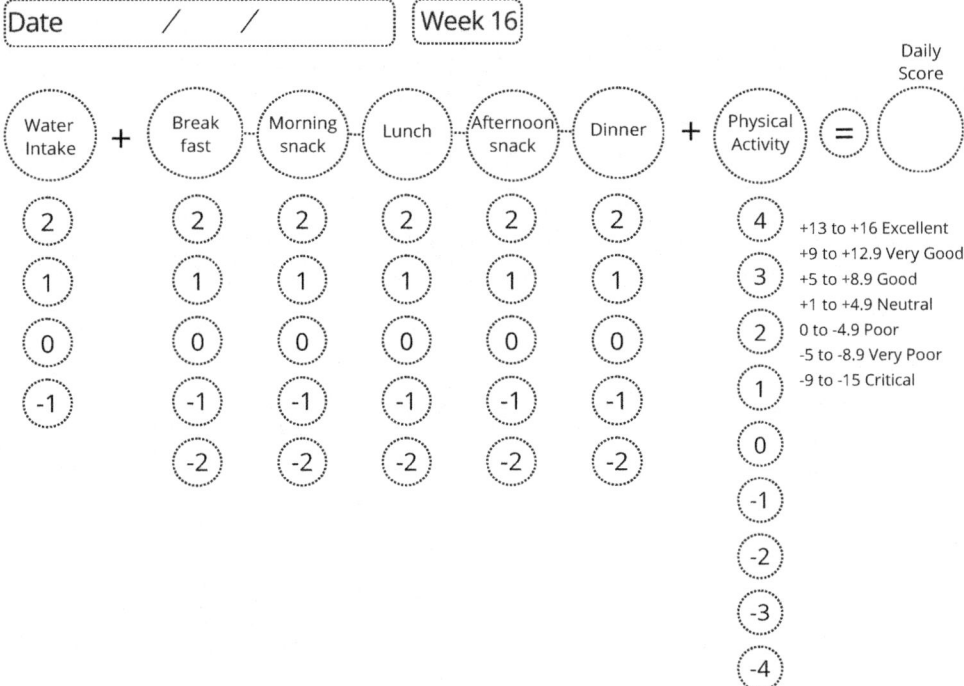

Date ___ / ___ / ___   Week 16

Daily Score

Water Intake + Break fast · Morning snack · Lunch · Afternoon snack · Dinner + Physical Activity = ◯

Water Intake	Breakfast	Morning snack	Lunch	Afternoon snack	Dinner	Physical Activity	
2	2	2	2	2	2	4	+13 to +16 Excellent
1	1	1	1	1	1	3	+9 to +12.9 Very Good
0	0	0	0	0	0	2	+5 to +8.9 Good
-1	-1	-1	-1	-1	-1	1	+1 to +4.9 Neutral
	-2	-2	-2	-2	-2	0	0 to -4.9 Poor
						-1	-5 to -8.9 Very Poor
						-2	-9 to -15 Critical
						-3	
						-4	

End of Week 16 – Weekly Summary

Congratulations on making it this far! Sixteen weeks of commitment, growth, and consistency — that's a major achievement. But remember: this isn't the end. It's the beginning of a healthier, more intentional life. To keep building on your progress, there's also the 6-Month Journal — a streamlined version without the theory, designed for those who already know the method and want to stay consistent. Keep going. The best is still ahead of you.

If this method has helped you, even in a small way, consider leaving a review. Your feedback can inspire others to begin their own journey — and it means the world to those of us who created this with care and purpose.

Weekly Summary Graph

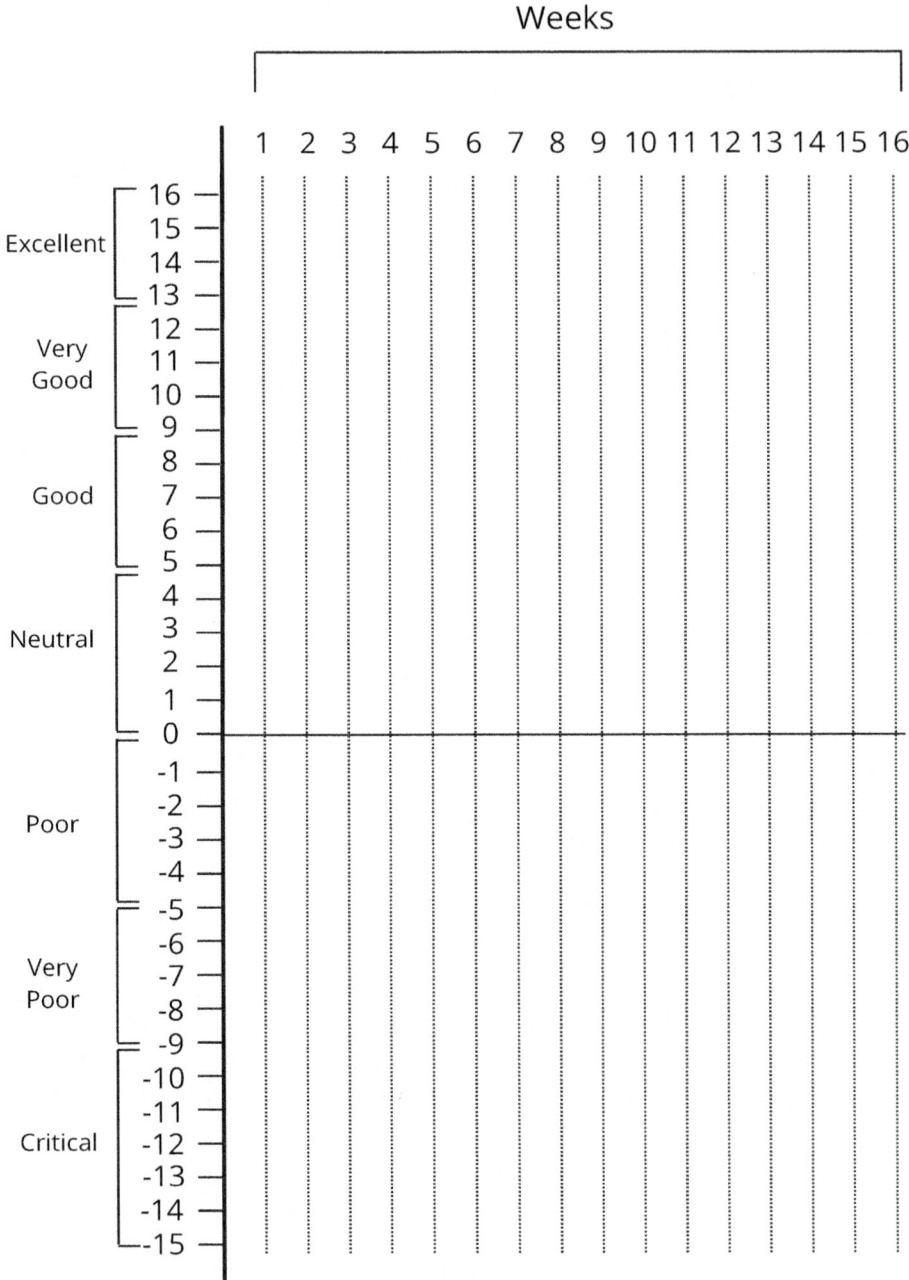

Place a dot at the average score for each week.
If you'd like, you can then connect the dots.

Printed in Dunstable, United Kingdom

76303461R00080